THE WORKING MOM'S HANDBOOK

THE
WORKING
MOM'S
HANDBOOK

A Survival Guide for Returning
to Work after Having a Baby

ALI VELEZ ALDERFER

ROCKRIDGE
PRESS

For general information on our other products and services or to obtain technical support, please contact our Customer Care Department within the United States at (866) 744-2665, or outside the United States at (510) 253-0500.

Rockridge Press publishes its books in a variety of electronic and print formats. Some content that appears in print may not be available in electronic books, and vice versa.

Interior and Cover Designer: Regina Stadnik
Photo Art Director/Art Manager: Sara Feinstein
Editor: Morgan Shanahan and Anne Lowrey
Production Editor: Ashley Polikoff

All illustrations used under license from iStock.com and Shutterstock.com

Author photo courtesy of A. Justin Alderfer

ISBN: Print 978-1-64739-635-0 | eBook 978-1-64739-636-7
R0

For Justin and Rafael, who inspire me every day. I love you both more than pizza. (But it's close.)

And for all the working moms out there—whether you're working to feed your family or to feed your soul—I see you.

CONTENTS

INTRODUCTION

When I arrived at my office on my first day back at work after my son was born, I discovered an outpouring of text messages from my incredible friends, most of them working moms who had already lived through their first day back. The messages of support, "You've got this!" and "Have a great day—your little guy is so loved and cared for right now," got me through that very tough day. And then came the next day (and weeks . . . and months). I didn't know what to do with the mixed bag of emotions I was carrying with me, and I was wholly unprepared for the tug-of-war that I was about to enter between my working life and my home life.

As I set out to write this book, I wanted to create the road map I wished I had been given to help me navigate the emotions, politics, and logistics of being a working mom. Every article I saw online basically just said, "You're doing great, mama!" . . . but I didn't believe it. It felt like empty encouragement from Instagram influencers selling the idea that all moms are great moms—just by virtue of being one—and deserve bubble baths, pedicures, and wine. What was I doing wrong to feel like I wasn't succeeding enough at home or at work? Plus, who has time for pedicures? And bubble baths are nice and all, but I don't really feel like having to get on my hands and knees to scrub the tub clean for a few minutes of "relaxation." Self-care sounded an awful lot like chores.

I decided it was time to write honestly about what it means to be a parent who works. I talked to a lot of working mothers, from all different work backgrounds and life experiences. This book is for everyone, from the retail associate to the CEO, from single parents carrying the load to couples with a live-in village of support. Every story helped inform what I hope will be a handy guidebook for navigating your own experience of working parenthood. I'm not a parenting expert. I'm just a working mom who tries to make the best choices for myself, my family, and my career every day.

After the birth of my son, I suffered from postpartum anxiety, which was exacerbated by the fact that I had to go back to work. As much as I loved my job before I became a mom,

I wanted more time to figure things out before I went back to it. But like a lot of moms, my family needed the income and health insurance my job provided. Eventually, I got back into the swing of things at work, and got more used to the idea of leaving my baby. Even then, I felt like I became invisible at work. I was having a hard time advancing my career while my childless peers were making upward strides. With the added expenses that come along with a new baby, my husband and I were both working so hard just to stay afloat that we weren't really getting to see our baby a whole lot. There was definitely a deficit in the "life" part of the work-life balance. The path we were on was unsustainable, especially when I felt so unsatisfied at work.

We decided it was time for a big change, and so we took a leap of faith in ourselves and our family. We sold our home in Los Angeles and left behind our jobs (mid-career!), our friends, and everything we knew, and moved to the suburbs outside of Atlanta. There we could afford, at least for a while, to be a one-income family while I figured out what was next for me. As it turns out, my next chapter was staying home with my 18-month-old in a town where I had no village, no community, and no lifeline.

It was tough. I loved having time with my son, but the days were long and lonely with my husband working long hours. After almost a year of not working (for the first time in my adult life), and getting my son acclimated to our new home, I was hungry for more. We found an amazing preschool for my son, who was now two years old, and, after dipping my toes back into the work space with some freelance editing from home, I managed to find a job that challenges me, offers great benefits for my family, and has clear opportunities for advancement. Yes, the anxiety was still there, and leaving my son when he was a toddler was just as hard as leaving him when he was a newborn, but it was also great to get back into the working world and feel a little more like myself.

At the beginning of this book's journey, I had it all figured out. I was able to manage my time between my full-time job, having a very active toddler at home, and making time for my marriage and myself. Between preschool, the help of a wonderful part-time babysitter, and a work schedule that allowed me to spend some afternoons with my family, I was still able to carve out writing time and even managed to be around for bedtime stories and snuggles. I was crushing this whole working-mom thing.

And then a funny thing happened on the way to the office. A global pandemic fell upon us and changed everything. I work in digital journalism and news, so my day job was by no means slowing down. I was still working full-time from home. And guess what? My book-writing deadlines didn't change either. But guess what did change? Suddenly, I was working two jobs from home with NO CHILDCARE. Preschool (and all schools) were closed—indefinitely. Self-isolation and quarantine rules did not include visits from our beloved babysitter.

Suddenly, like many parents across the globe, I was discovering what it looked like when everyday parenting was simply parenting in survival mode. Priorities were turned on their head. The whole world was upside down. And that anxiety? Still alive and well.

Somehow, we continue to survive. We make it work. I'm a mom. What choice do we have? In attempting to find things to be thankful for (I still have a job that provides income and health insurance, my family is safe and healthy, and I have a backyard for my three-year-old to run and play in that's safe from the rest of the world) in these trying and uncertain times, I felt a profound sense of gratitude for this book. As I wrote words of encouragement to new parents out there facing challenges I couldn't have imagined, it forced me to give myself a bit of grace in trying to do it all while most people are just trying to get through the day.

So, let's jump into this whole working-parent life thing, shall we? Think of this book as your cheerleader through the best times—when your hair is clean, you nailed that presentation at work, and still made it home for bath time and good night kisses—and also as your supportive "tough love" bestie through the harder days, when you feel like something's gotta give. There is tremendous pressure on parents to perfectly balance family and career, or "have it all." It may feel impossible, but it's not out of reach. Having it all just might look a little different from what you thought it would be.

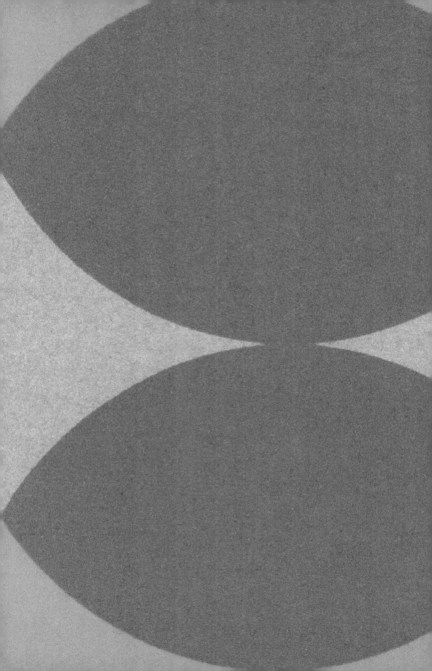

BABIES, BUSINESS, AND BOUNDARIES: PREPARING TO RETURN TO WORK

So, you're ready to go back to work. Or maybe you're not quite ready, but it's happening anyway. Either way, you are not alone. Whether you became a parent weeks ago (congrats!), or you are going back to work after an extended period of time staying home with your littles, it can be a bit overwhelming, but it can also be an incredibly beautiful and empowering time for you.

The choice to go back to work is not always the easiest one to make, so congratulate yourself on getting this far. Now take a deep breath, and let's get down to the business of getting back to business.

In this section, we're going to cover some of the more personal and emotional aspects of working parenthood. This is a time to take stock of your personal and professional priorities and how they may have shifted since that little stranger came into your life. You might find yourself more ambitious than ever to kick your career into high gear, or you may be a little less driven to put in the extra hours at work for that big promotion you previously thought you wanted, because you'd rather spend more time at home. It is totally normal and valid to swing in either direction. No matter how you're feeling, you've got this.

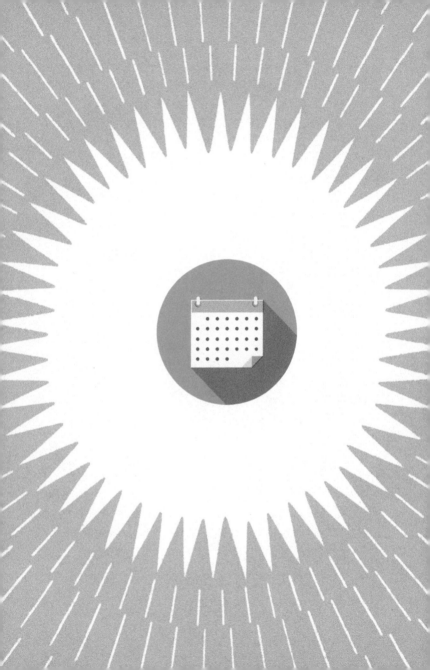

CHAPTER 1

What No One Really Tells You about Going Back to Work

Going back to work means different things to different parents. Most often, we think of the parents who are returning to a structured, 40-hour workweek in some type of office or corporate environment after taking time off based on their company's preestablished parental leave policy. But we can't forget the people who work nontraditional hours, take an hourly wage, work from home, own their own business, or are freelancers. And let's hear it for the parents who are on their feet all day in physically demanding jobs or working graveyard shifts.

No matter how and where you go to work, a job requires your time, energy, and attention, all of which have just become very precious commodities. Leaving your baby with someone else—whether that person is a relative (hooray for local grandparents!) or a virtual stranger you have put your faith in (take a deep breath, your tiny human will be so loved)—can be emotionally taxing and even a bit traumatic. But you know what? It can also be liberating and exciting. Nobody pulling at your boobs and spitting up in your hair! Adult conversations!

Part of "having it all" as a new mom means knowing your rights. Learning what you are entitled to in terms of job security and accommodations will help you protect yourself against being penalized for taking any sort of leave benefit offered by your employer (or by the Family and Medical Leave Act). Workplace logistics and politics can be super complicated, but I'm going to break it all down for you so you can replace a lot of that confusion and anxiety with confidence.

It's also time to get real about what motherhood and work means for you financially. There's a lot to think about in terms of cost-benefit strategies. How does the cost of your preferred method of childcare factor into your current income situation? Let's also not forget about the idea of emotional and mental health vs. financial health, and finding a balance in all the benefits and deficits that your current (or future) decisions might carry. It sounds daunting, but I wrote this book to help you map it all out, so you are ready to make the best, most-informed choices for you and your family!

Here is a list of some things to think about (and be honest with yourself about) in terms of your goals and expectations, before diving into this section:

- What are your immediate goals and expectations upon returning to your job?

- What are some of your long-term professional goals?

- Are any of these goals and expectations different now that you are a parent? (Which is totally normal!)

- Are you open to a career or job change that fits your new lifestyle?

NAVIGATING YOUR CHILDCARE OPTIONS

Finding the right childcare for your family is probably one of the most important, and most anxiety-ridden, decisions you'll have to make. But make no mistake—if you want to go back to work, it's something you need to think about sooner rather than way too late. If you're reading this book, you're most likely expecting or already on parental leave. Without being overly dramatic, I'm here to tell you that if you have not already made childcare arrangements, you need to get on that NOW.

This is something I wish someone had told me when I was pregnant, as I found myself in a panic just a few weeks out from the end of my leave, when every single day care I called had a waitlist for infants. I was told by more than one provider that the waiting list for newborns or infants was 18 months. Yup, you read that right. Even if I had placed my name on a day care waiting list the day I peed on that stick, I'd still have to wait another nine months after he was born to get him a spot. How does that even make sense when, after 18 months, a child is no longer considered a newborn or an infant? THAT IS A FULL-ON TODDLER.

I was fortunate that my mom was able to fly cross-country to come and stay for the first few weeks after my return to work, and in the meantime, we were able to find a local in-home day care that we could afford. But I know not everyone has a family member who can step in and save the day, so it's time to start asking yourself some really big questions.

Only you (and your partner, if applicable) know what kind of childcare option is the best for your family. Once you've decided on relatives vs. nannies vs. day care (and any other option or combo platter of the above), it's time to ask the tough questions about what "having it all" means to you.

How much time are you willing to spend away from your child? How much do you need to work in order to pay for childcare, and is one parent essentially working just to cover the costs of care? This is definitely a time to reflect and take a good, honest look at your priorities—without judgment. What do you need in order to be able to go after your career goals, but still have the time (and the bandwidth) to spend with your baby? Does your job often require that you take your work home with you? If you're working in order to get out of the house a bit and earn some extra money (because diapers don't pay for themselves), are you willing to consider a career shift into something less ambitious and demanding, that you can leave behind when you clock out? If you're working toward a certain career goal, are you willing to accept that your baby will be spending a great deal of their awake time with someone else? (Now is a good time to remember that nothing can replace the connection your baby has to you. You are imprinted on each other for life.)

You don't have to have all of the answers right now. But it's time to start asking the questions.

Here's how some other moms across the country answered these questions for themselves:

Coby, an attorney from Sacramento, CA: *"Given the cost, it was not practical for my husband to have a full-time job. We decided to have him work part-time from home. I had to learn I literally cannot give everything 100 percent. I am a perfectionist and it kills me still. But I have to just switch it off or I'd never be able to be there for my family."*

Liza, a part-time server from Annapolis, MD: *"It made sense for us to take a bit of a financial hit for me to not work a ton of hours. I loved being at home, but it was challenging. I didn't realize how much of my self-worth was attached to being fiscally independent and bringing income to my family. I had to remind myself (and my husband at times) that cleaning the toilets, doing all the laundry, the shopping, some cooking, and all the other things to make a home—AND raising my daughter to be a happy, loving, kind, well-adjusted person—were just as valuable, if not more so. Paying others to take care of my daughter was a big deal since I was home to do that. So dates and other grown-up types of fun events were at a minimum."*

Ashley, a marketing manager from Los Angeles, CA: *"With my first, I felt a lot of guilt that she was spending more time with her teacher than me. On weekends, I felt a need to make every single moment* special and fun, which is exhausting in the long run. But now, I'm so happy that my kids are in day care. They (and we) have made lifelong friends and they are so socially adept."

Kristina, a paralegal from Denver, CO: *"I was able to work from home on Mondays and Tuesday mornings. My husband travels for work, so when he's not traveling, he's working from home. We were able to find a nanny for our daughter at a very affordable rate. With me working from home a day and a half per week, and my husband making his own schedule, we were able to keep the nanny hours to about 20 hours per week."*

THINGS THAT ARE OKAY

Getting back into an old routine when you have a completely new life is hard. You're going back to an environment that has stayed the same, while you have changed in ways you can't even describe. So, yeah. It's going to get weird. THAT'S OKAY. You know what else is okay? Giving yourself a break and handling it all in your own way.

Here are some other things that are totally, completely, 100 percent okay:

- Being super anxious about going back to work

- Being really excited about getting dressed up and going to work. (That's right, both feelings are TOTALLY NORMAL AND OKAY.)

- Being psyched about GROWN-UP CONVERSATIONS WITH GROWN-UPS!

- Crying at work, or on the way to work, or after work . . .

- Being devastated (and, yes, maybe crying) over spilled breast milk

- Clocking in and out and doing what's expected of you, and nothing more

- Not taking work home with you

- Staying late because your work is important to you. (This doesn't mean your family isn't important! Both things can be true.)

- Talking about your baby a lot

- Not talking about your baby at all

- Being honest with yourself and your supervisor about what kind of workload you can handle

- Wishing you could be home with your kiddo

- Being grateful for time away from your kiddo

- Still wearing maternity pants or maxi dresses to work because your body is still recovering from CARRYING AND BIRTHING A HUMAN

- Taking time to go somewhere private and pump as frequently as you need to. (In fact, it's more than okay, it's your right.)

- Speaking up when someone says something rude about you doing any of these things or asks you an inappropriate question about your boobs

- Crying some more

- Calling your child's caregiver to check in and see how they are doing

- Enjoying your commute and going to the bathroom at work, because ALONE TIME is sacred

- Peeing yourself a little when someone makes you laugh, when you sneeze, or just randomly. (Sorry, not sorry—it's going to happen.)

Set Your Budget

Babies are expensive. It's shocking how much your diaper budget is in reality vs. what you imagined. How can such a teeny-tiny creature fill so many diapers in a day? (Or honestly, in an hour!) But the prices of diapers and wipes have got NOTHING on how much childcare can set you back. Luckily, there are tools to help you figure out how to determine what you can and should be paying based on your current financial situation.

According to a comprehensive study done by Care.com, the average annual price of childcare ($9,589) is higher than the yearly cost of in-state college tuition ($9,410). And that's for in-center care. The average cost of childcare at home is a whopping $28,354. Yeah. I'm going to let you just sit with that and breathe for a minute.

If you're trying to figure out what kind of care you're looking for AND can afford, you're going to have to do a little math. Whether you're trying to figure out what salary you have to make in order to afford the care you want, OR what kind of care you can swing based on your current or expected income, there are a few tools and formulas that can help.

The US Department of Health and Human Services (HHS.gov) suggests that the cost of care should not exceed 10 percent of your annual household income. This figure, however, doesn't necessarily account for any or all of your other household expenses. So, to get a clearer picture, you can use one of several online calculators, like the one from ChildCareAware.org, to make a monthly budget based on your family's total income and expenses.

And there's help, too! Don't forget about federal and state tax credits for child and dependent care. You should also look into your (or your partner's) health care plan to see if you are eligible for a Flexible Spending Account (FSA) or a Health Spending Account (HSA) and if childcare costs qualify under those programs.

Get Those Expectations in Check

Okay, now that you've figured out how much you are willing and, more important, able to pay for childcare, you can make some solid choices about what your preferences are. Nannies tend to be on the more expensive side, so you might be sacrificing your time in exchange for one-on-one attention and care. Does your budget allow for a full-time nanny? If so, for how many hours are you okay leaving your baby with them—or, on the flip side, how many hours do you need to put in at work to afford it? Would you need or expect this person to also help around the house with things like cleaning and cooking, and does that add an extra expense?

If you don't mind your baby having a little company and you don't want to break the bank for private care, you could consider a nanny share, in which you and another family would split the cost of a caregiver who would look after both children together, or on separate part-time shifts. If you want your child to be socialized a bit more, day care is definitely a more cost-effective option (and a great way for your child to make some friends with kids around the same age). Plus, day care is not a one-size-fits-all situation.

Aside from the bigger care centers, you can opt for an in-home day care. These providers usually only care for a small group of children (typically around six), and have at least two or three adults present. In these cases, you get a really nice blend of socialization and individual attention. And there's always the option of someone you know—grandparents, friends, neighbors, or a combo of members in your village—who wants to help out. This can be a very personal decision, so you need to follow your gut, and be prepared to set some boundaries and expectations with your chosen caregiver.

As you make your choices on how and where you want your child cared for, there are a lot of variables to consider. What are your goals and expectations for care? In other words, what do you need from your provider to make you feel comfortable with leaving your child in their care? What kind of updates do you need on your baby's day and any milestones?

The first few weeks, I asked my son's caregiver to send me photos. It made missing him during the day a little easier (and, honestly, sometimes a little tougher). You can absolutely let your provider know about any preferences you have about feeding, diapering, and the like. And it's okay to have a lot of questions about their policies on everything from redirection for undesired behavior to nap schedules to emergency preparedness. There is no question too big or too small.

Having an open and honest discussion with your parents or your in-laws can be especially tricky. These are the people who raised you and your partner—and will remind you of that fact every chance they get. Yes, they have experience. Yes, they love your child. But a lot has changed since they were in the hot seat, and it's okay to let them know how you want things handled.

Even if your family members are not going to be your primary source of childcare while you're working, now is a great time to set up some simple ground rules for any relatives who will be spending time in your home and around your baby. Some of these issues may include access to the baby and whether you are open to unsolicited advice. Sorry, cousin Lisa, please keep your slight head cold as far away as possible. And yes, Dad, I know they didn't have Purell back in your day and everyone survived, but if you don't clean your hands, you don't get to hold the baby. (Thanks for playing.) You can also use these conversations to be clear about what you do need help with. I promise you, people will step up in the little ways you need the most if you just ask.

This is also the time to have a heart-to-heart with your partner about how you want to handle any issues with each other's parents, and how to deal with the inevitable

Grandparent Wars. Having a plan for grandparental jealousy will save you a lot of stress if and when it comes up—especially if one set of grandparents has a geographical advantage over the other. Talk it out and make a plan. Maybe you make an agreement that you each will deal with your own parents for the tough stuff, or maybe you want to have a big family meeting to get everyone on the same page at once. Develop a code word or phrase with your partner when you need to take a sidebar. You know your family dynamic best; just make sure that you and your partner have each other's backs so you can handle who gets to be called Pop-Pop vs. Nanno as a unified front.

BUT I WORK FROM HOME. I DON'T NEED CHILDCARE, RIGHT?

Newborns sleep a lot. This is true. But you know what else is true? They need constant attention. And they are tiny, exhausting creatures that eat and poop A LOT. Working from home presents some unique opportunities and challenges for a new parent. Depending on how demanding or time-sensitive your work is, working from home affords you the ability to be able to nurse your baby throughout the day, which is helpful if you've chosen to exclusively breastfeed. You also get some quality snuggle time to break up the day. But in most cases, it's a lot more work and stress to divide your energy and focus between your two very important jobs.

You need to really assess how Baby's needs fit into your work schedule and emotional and mental health. Maybe your work hours are flexible and you can spend time doting on Baby during the day and doing your boss business at night. When does that leave time for you to rest and recharge? What if Baby starts crying when you're in the middle of a conference call or in the thick of a rush to meet a deadline?

In most cases, having a caregiver around (at least part of the time) helps ease the burden of you trying to be everything to everyone all the time. Repeat after me: childcare is self-care.

Now, once more for the people in the back: CHILDCARE IS SELF-CARE!

WHAT TO EXPECT WHEN YOU'RE EXPECTING TO LEAVE YOUR BABY WITH SOMEONE ELSE

Leaving your baby is going to be hard. There's no way around that. But, if you have a childcare provider that you trust (whether it's a nanny, a day care, or a relative), it will get easier. You'll just need to set some very clear expectations up front.

The same way your boss has clear expectations and goals for you when you come to work, you need to remember that in this situation, YOU are the boss and the caregiver is working for you (yes, even if it's your own mother). You can be grateful for the help while also asking for what you want and need in terms of your child's care. When someone is doing you a favor—like a grandparent watching the baby FOR FREE—it can feel a little awkward to "lay down the law," but it can be even more awkward if you have to miss your big work presentation because Nana wanted to make a Target run before coming over.

Once you've set some realistic expectations with your caregiver regarding the feeding schedule, allergies, photos and updates, and whether cooking and cleaning are part of the equation (if you have someone to help in your home), you can rest knowing that your child is going to be well taken care of. Still, there is bound to be a roller coaster of emotions that come with leaving your baby with someone else.

There will be tears. I'm not just talking about your baby here. It's totally normal to feel a sense of loss or sadness after handing off your little angel. You've been bonding with this perfect little person and separating is hard! It doesn't seem possible, but I swear it does get easier eventually.

Guilt is a garbage emotion, but a very real one nonetheless. I would tell you not to feel guilty, but that would be a waste of my time and yours. What I can tell you is to remind yourself of all the reasons why you made the exact right choices that brought you to this place. Trust in yourself that you are absolutely doing the best thing for yourself and your family. And get ready for the one-two punch of eventually starting to feel really good, excited, or relieved to hand off your baby, and then BOOM!

Return of the Guilt! The Guilt Strikes Back! The Self-Shame Awakens! Resist the guilt and shame. You and Baby are doing fine.

The one thing I was not expecting to experience when I left my son—first with my mom, and then at a small day care—and that came over me like a tidal wave, was *jealousy*. I was so afraid that my baby would wind up bonding with my mom and his day care provider, and I actually thought it was possible for him to love them more than me. I was jealous of the time they got to spend holding him, feeding him, and watching him change, day after day. I was irrationally terrified that he would laugh for the first time and I would miss it. I mean, my mom is pretty damn funny.

Of course, what I discovered (and you will, too), is that as cliché as it sounds, love multiplies. I was grateful for the love and care that my son not only received but felt for his Nana, and also for the wonderful woman that took care of him in her home. It made me happy to hear of all the discoveries he was making at day care, knowing that he had all of these amazing women in his life who loved him so. And none of that took away anything from our bond. Babies always know their parents. Always.

It can be hard to step outside yourself and recognize the difference between the "baby blues" and clinical post-partum depression (PPD) or postpartum anxiety (PPA). Circumstantial depression, such as adjustment disorder, can affect anyone going through a serious life transition. If you think you might be experiencing PPD or PPA, or you feel like something is just not right (you know yourself better than anyone), it is absolutely worth reaching out to your physician or therapist for help or guidance.

Symptoms of postpartum depression and anxiety typically start showing up in the first four weeks after giving birth, although for some women, changes in mood and behavior can start late into the third trimester of pregnancy.

Symptoms can include, but are not limited to:

- Feelings of emptiness and hopelessness

- Irritability, anxiousness, and guilt

- Feelings of exhaustion and severe tiredness

- Feelings of tension

- Loss of interest and energy

- Inability to concentrate or remember details

- Suicidal thoughts or attempts of suicide

- Disturbing thoughts or images you can't shake

- Changes in appetite—eating too much or too little

- Physical symptoms—aches and pains, cramps, headaches, digestive issues, breast tenderness, bloating

- Mood swings

- Panic attacks

- Sleep disturbances, such as sleeping too much or too little, and insomnia

If you are struggling and need help, reach out to a trusted health care provider such as your ob-gyn, midwife, family physician, or therapist.

The Patient Health Questionnaire (PHQ-9) is also a helpful guide for self-assessment (but not meant to substitute for professional medical advice or treatment). Read about it and access the questionnaire at ncbi.nlm.nih.gov /pmc/articles/PMC1495268.

If you are in crisis, you can call the National Suicide Prevention Lifeline at 1-800-273-8255. You can also text HOME to 741741 to reach the Crisis Text Line for immediate help.

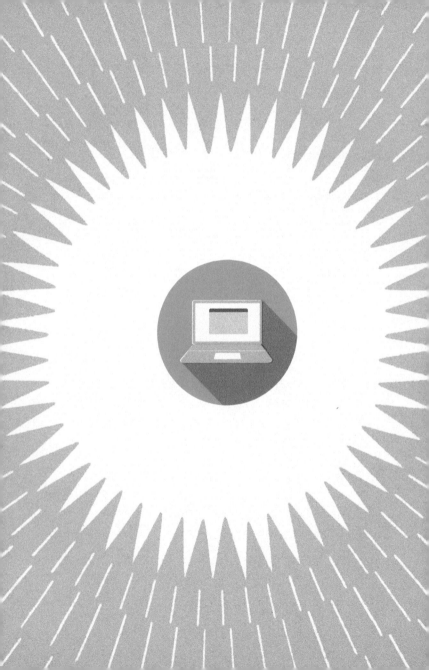

CHAPTER 2

Picking Up Where You Left Off . . . ish

On my first day back to work, it felt good to be all showered and dressed up with somewhere to go, but everything else was difficult. My mom practically had to pry the baby out of my arms. I was able to keep it together for most of the day at work, until a colleague asked me how I was holding up and I just started to cry in the middle of the office. I contemplated whether the work I was doing was "important enough" to justify being away from my tiny baby all day.

One week later, I was driving home from a really great, productive day at work when I realized I hadn't felt sad that day about being away from my baby. And then I immediately cried because I felt guilty. Again, I thought about my priorities. My job wasn't changing the world, but I knew I needed to keep doing it. Practically, my family needed my income and the health benefits my job offered. Personally, I needed to be doing something creative, and to be around people who challenged and inspired me, in order to be the best version of myself at home. The sadness and guilt still came in waves, but I did my best to make every moment count, both at work and at home.

TL;DR: Going back to work can be both wonderful and terrible, and it's okay to have complicated feelings.

PRIORITIES—THE WAY THEY WERE

It goes without saying that once that tiny human arrives, your priorities change pretty fast. Remember when showering regularly, eating three square meals a day, and watching your favorite TV shows the night they aired was a thing? In the early days after birth, a lot of self-care goes out the window as we focus on our number one objective: keep Baby alive. Secondary priorities include keeping up with Baby's input (So. Many. Feedings.) and output (So. Many. Diapers.), trying to make them smile, and taking a thousand pictures an hour at the cost of our own hygiene, rest, and comfort.

Take all of that change, add in a dash of attachment and a sprinkle of exhaustion, and it's only natural that some of your big-picture priorities might be shifting as well. And you're not the only one. Your partner may also be having conflicting feelings about work and time at home and money and sleep and ALL THE THINGS.

This is really a time to reflect and have a serious conversation about career and family goals, and what makes sense financially and logically now. Maybe you are more motivated than ever to move your career forward. If so, go after it! Or you could find yourself having some trepidation about the demands of your job. Does that promotion you were chasing before Baby involve more travel or late nights at the office than you want to put in now? Have you and your partner discussed whether one of you has a "higher priority" career in terms of income, status, or passion? How much does it matter if one of you is more passionate about your work than the other? Which job gets you that good health insurance, which is more important now than ever? These questions are all things to keep in mind as you make your plans to either return to your previous job or maybe make a shift to something that fulfills your desire to work and allows you to have the work-life balance you're looking for.

There's no one-size-fits-all answer to the questions. Like so many of us, your work has probably been a part of your identity for most of your adult life. There are certain expectations that come with that. And now you're a parent, which is a whole other identity in itself, with its own set of rules and expectations. The tricky part is finding a way to honor all the things that make you who you are: your work, your relationships, your family, and your dreams. You're a complex being with complex wants and needs!

IDENTIFYING PRIORITY SHIFTS

You doing okay? Remember, it's normal to have some mixed feelings. Now that you're a parent, you're probably remembering that time you judged—if even for a second—the woman who drank her coffee while her toddler was having a meltdown in the grocery store. Suddenly feeling flooded with empathy? Or maybe you're laughing about that time you said you'd never use a pacifier, while you wipe off the one that just fell on the floor and put it back in your baby's mouth. Whatever. Everything changes when it's your turn.

It's gut check time. Are you relating to your friend who decided to stay home with her baby because the finances of childcare didn't make sense? Or are you totally getting why your coworker couldn't wait to get back to work, even if it meant practically handing her check directly to the nanny or day care so she didn't lose the momentum she was building professionally? Or maybe you just need to get out there and do your work to feel creatively and intellectually whole? Are you itching to start something new, maybe feeling inspired by the new life you've created?

Make two lists on the next page: Your priorities and goals before you had your baby vs. now. Is there any overlap? What's the same? What's drastically different? What conversations do you need to have with your partner or your boss as a result of these insights?

BEFORE BABY	AFTER BABY

PERSONAL	PROFESSIONAL

RECONCILING WHAT'S CHANGED SINCE MOTHERHOOD (AND WHAT HASN'T)

When it comes to shifting priorities and goals, there is no right answer; you just have to find the right balance for your family. Here's what some other moms I talked to had to say about their experiences:

Cassandra, a senior producer of video programming from Woodstock, GA: "My priorities definitely changed. My mindset is family first. I work to provide for my family. I used to not mind staying late for meetings, etc. but now when I am off the clock I want to be off the clock. I want to head home so I can snuggle with my little guy all night. I get irritated when my boss contacts me off-hours—it makes me feel like he doesn't respect my work-life balance. I try not to be on email or connected when I am off-hours. I want to get in, do my job, and get home."

Yeneir, a teacher from Miami, FL: "I had more ambition, more expectations, and I had more demands on myself. I wanted my daughter to know that you can be a mother, a wife, and a professional, and be great at all three without sacrificing one or the other."

Courtney, a structural engineer from Beaufort, SC:
*"I think I became less ambitious as time went on.
At first, I felt like I could make it work—that I would
just pull up my bootstraps and show them all what
a woman was capable of . . . that I could "have it
all." After a few months, I realized I couldn't be the
mother I wanted to be AND the career woman
I wanted to be. I had to be more careful about my
decisions to try to do only things that would bring
the MOST benefit, as my time was limited. I would
be aware that I wasn't performing to the level
I wanted to, but also knew that I couldn't if I wanted
to make it home for bedtime, or—as my child got
older—karate or baseball. I don't think it's possible
to be the very best at my career AND be the mom
I want to be. So I find myself saying, 'This is the best
I can do,' and trying to be okay with not achieving
everything at work that I want to."*

Taysha, a graphic designer from Los Angeles, CA:
*"I always knew I'd have to go back to work. Staying
at home just wasn't an option for me, and, frankly,
I enjoy working and the financial stability it brings
to my family. I was happy to get back to work,
seeing coworkers and friends, but also sad because
I missed my baby. I really thought I was going
to miss something spectacular. My husband*

would tell me, "He doesn't even know you were gone . . ." My company is really great at making sure a work-home-life balance is a priority. I think I was the one who had to change my attitude and expectations, as I've been in the corporate world for so long without a family. Even though I was happy with the status quo, the changing environment within my department made it necessary to take on a senior leadership role."

BRINGING RIGHTS TO LIGHT: DOWNSTREAM SETBACKS AND HOW TO AVOID THEM

Although the United States may be woefully behind the rest of the developed world in terms of paid parental leave, the Family and Medical Leave Act (FMLA) does offer 12 weeks of unpaid, job-protected time off for most new parents (including foster and adoptive parents) in the workplace. In general, private employers with 50 or more employees are covered by the law. To qualify, you must have been working for your employer for at least 12 months. Those 12 months do not need to be consecutive; so if you work on a seasonal shift, you may still be eligible as long as you have worked for 12 months overall, and as long as there hasn't been a break in service of seven years or more. The FMLA also has special rules and consider-ations for some nontraditional work schedules, such as airline flight crew employees. Make sure you know your rights as they pertain to your specific job situation.

The FMLA is there to protect you and your job. The law requires that when you return, your employer must restore you to your same position—or one that is nearly identical—with the same pay, benefits, and a comparable schedule. So it doesn't matter if Julie the temp did a great job covering for you and everybody loved her; you still get to have your job back.

So yes, in theory, everything should be the same when you get back to work. But everything is not the same. Your life has changed, maybe your priorities, too, and that's okay—and protected by the law. Yes, there are laws protecting your right to have a safe, clean place (and the time) to pump milk in privacy at work, if you are still nursing or pumping. We will dive deeper into this topic in the next section of the book.

The most important way to protect yourself and your job is to know your rights. For more information on what you're entitled to, how to apply for the FMLA, and guidance on what to do if you feel like you're experiencing discrimination after you return to work from leave, visit DOL.gov /agencies/whd/fmla, or Benefits.gov/benefit/5895.

MOMMY TRACKING: WHAT IS IT AND HOW FAST CAN WE MAKE THAT TERM GO AWAY?

Believe it or not, the "mommy track" is a real thing—but a smart parent like you does not have to subscribe to it. The concept of "mommy tracking" is the idea that there is (or should be) an easier, less demanding career path for mothers in the workplace that sacrifices opportunities for advancement in place of more flexibility and time off for family issues. The mommy track could be seen as a positive compromise for some women who CHOOSE to take a step back at work, but it's often a decision that's silently made by an employer who assumes it's the best choice for everyone.

Only YOU get to decide what's right for you in terms of your career trajectory. You'll probably notice that nobody ever assumes or suggests that new dads would want to be on a similar "daddy track," so what gives? Oftentimes, lowering demands and expectations of new moms at work isn't even done with malice or as a "punishment" for taking time off; sometimes it's just a blanket assumption about what new moms need without actually conferring with the new mom.

Side note: A year after I had come back to work from having my son, I was struggling to advance. Any movement I was making at work was a lateral move, while others around me were being promoted and given bigger opportunities and challenges. When I reached out to my HR representative to discuss my concerns, this person, who was supposed to be there to support my needs in the workplace, actually made a joke—in writing—directly suggesting that I wasn't being promoted because I had taken some time off "for a very good reason!" This was A WHOLE YEAR after I had come back from leave. The leave that was freely offered to me and every other employee (male or female) of the company. I was "mommy tracked" before I ever knew what that meant.

So, yeah. This is a real—although mostly unspoken—issue, and the only way to combat it is to speak up. Don't let the choice be made for you. You actually do get a say.

To avoid any confusion, try to set up a meeting with your direct manager or supervisor before your scheduled return date. If meeting in person is not possible, set up a phone or video call, or even a back-and-forth email discussion (bonus: with email, you have records of everything discussed). This is a great time to let your supervisor know what your goals are and what you are willing to give in terms of hours and workflow. You can work with them to set clear goals and expectations on both sides, so that you can feel confident that when you return to the job, you're returning to the job you want. And they can be confident in knowing that they can trust you to handle your previous workload and more, if that's what you want.

If you do want to step back a little—for example, you want the job security but need to lighten the load a bit—that's still your choice to make and it's totally okay to ask for what you need.

It's all up to you. And nobody knows what you need and what you are capable of better than you do.

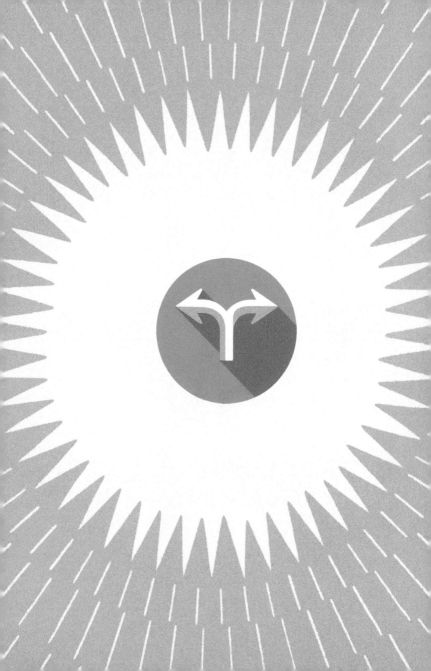

CHAPTER 3

Career Pathing/ Development: Where Does Your Career Go from Here?

N ow that you've got childcare covered and a sense of how to approach those first few days back, let's talk bigger picture about your career. Maybe you're one of the lucky ones who already has a job you love, so going back is a seamless transition. Maybe your employer provides on-site childcare, so working extra hours isn't as much of an issue. But perhaps, like the vast majority of working parents in the United States, you're still building your career and starting a family complicates that effort. It's time for you to lay the groundwork for your success, in whatever way success is defined by you moving forward.

What follows are some questions I wish someone had asked me to consider as I returned to work. Give yourself some time to evaluate each one, and be honest with your responses. You can mentally answer them and use them as prompts for a bit of a gut check with yourself. You may find it easier to journal your answers, or simply write out the responses you most want to get clear on. If that's the case, keep a pen and pad of paper nearby.

If you're feeling overwhelmed by all the questions, that's okay! Feel free to skip ahead to the next section and revisit when you're ready.

COMPATIBILITY TEST 1:
YOUR JOB AND YOUR FAMILY

1. How much time do you want or expect to spend at home with your family?

2. How important is it for you to be around for dinnertime and your baby's bedtime routine?

3. How important to you are your specific job and role?

4. Ideally, how many hours a week are you willing and able to spend at work?

5. How flexible do you need your job to be in terms of doctor visits (babies have a LOT of those in the first year) and potential family emergencies?

6. How important or vital is your income to the family's overall budget?

7. What accommodations will you need from your employer in order to go back to work (clean, private pumping area; unlimited sick or personal days; the ability to work from home when needed; etc.)?

8. What are the top priorities and benefits of going back to work (personal fulfillment, health insurance, financial stability, personal and professional work relationships)?

9. What are your immediate goals in terms of your job and where you left off when you took leave?

10. How comfortable do you feel when it comes to discussing personal and family matters with your direct manager?

11. How compatible is your childcare provider's schedule with your work schedule?

12. Do you feel supported in your workplace by coworkers and colleagues, management, and human resources?

13. Do you feel supported at home in your transition back to the working world?

COMPATIBILITY TEST 2:
YOUR CAREER AND YOUR FAMILY

1. What are your long-term career goals and ambitions?

2. Where would you like to be after your first year back?

3. What are your long-term goals and ideals as a parent?

4. What would you say is the most important factor in your path to career advancement and longevity (passion for the work, financial gains, personal drive and ambition, setting an example for your children, etc.)?

5. Did taking maternity leave set you back in your path at all in terms of missed opportunities, advancements in office policy, or technology, among other things?

6. What accommodations do you need at home in order to feel supported and successful in your career (home office space, extra childcare help from family, moral support from your partner, etc.)?

7. What steps do you need to take right away in order to prove to yourself and your employer that you are ready for all of your previous responsibilities or more?

8. How much time can you realistically expect or hope to be able to spend at home with your family?

9. What, if any, career perks will help foster your desired work-life balance (generous paid vacation policy, on-site childcare)?

10. What sacrifices are you willing to make in order to meet career expectations and milestones?

11. What sacrifices are you unwilling to make for your career and your family?

COMPATIBILITY TEST 3: YOUR JOB AND YOUR CAREER

1. Does your current job offer a pathway to your ultimate career goals?

2. If your job is not directly related to or in service of your eventual career aspirations,

what are ways in which you can make the most of your current situation (opportunities for networking, banking enough money to eventually take a risk in pursuing your dream career from scratch, building a certain skill set to enhance your resume)?

3. How long have you been at your current job?

4. Do you feel there is room for advancement in your current role?

5. Do you feel that taking leave was a setback, or are you coming back recharged and ready to push forward?

6. What are your short-term plans to make your transition back to work as seamless as possible?

7. What are your long-term plans to reach your ultimate career goals?

8. How do you define success in your desired career (job title, salary, professional reputation, creating or building your own business, retiring early)?

9. What sacrifices do you anticipate having to make in service of those ambitions?

MOVING ON UP!

Now that you're starting to have a clearer picture of what you want and need from your career, you can start setting yourself up for success—whatever that looks like to you. You've taken stock of your priorities and figured out what the ideal work-life balance is for you. That's a huge step. Now, how can you move toward advancing your career with so much on your plate? You absolutely have the power to succeed at work and at home. It's a balancing act, but a beautiful one when it all comes together.

I find routines and schedules to be extremely helpful. If you need a bit of structure to keep yourself on target, try mapping out what a typical day, week, or month might look like for you. Then, if there are any glaring deficits, such as not seeing your child at all on Tuesdays, you can make adjustments or find ways to make up time.

Honestly, there would be no way for me to get this book done AND see my family, all on top of my day job, if I didn't have it all scheduled. (And if I didn't have help.)

Here's an example of two typical days in a row with my current schedule:

Wednesday

4:30 a.m.–6:00 a.m.	wake up, get ready, commute to day job
6:00 a.m.–2:30 p.m.	day job (husband wakes up toddler, gets him to preschool)
2:30 p.m.–3:30 p.m.	commute home (babysitter picks up toddler from preschool)
3:30 p.m.–5:30 p.m.	book-writing
5:30 p.m.–6:30 p.m.	relieve babysitter, make dinner for toddler, eat, play, love
6:30 p.m.–7:30 p.m.	bath and bedtime routine: brushing teeth, putting on pj's, reading stories, all the hugs (both parents).
7:30 p.m.–9:30 / 10:00 p.m.	dinner and catching up with husband, maybe watch some TV
10:00 / 10:30 p.m.	sleep

Thursday

4:30 a.m.–6:00 a.m.	wake up, get ready, commute to day job
6:00 a.m.–2:30 p.m.	day job (husband wakes up toddler, gets him to preschool)
2:30 p.m.–3:15 p.m.	pick up toddler from preschool (yay!), go home
3:15 p.m.–5:00 p.m.	go on adventure or spend quality time with toddler (this activity can be a trip to the library, doing errands, going to the park, or playtime at home!)
OR 3:15 p.m.–5:00 p.m.	have a snack date (Dunkin' Donuts!) and then take toddler to gymnastics
5:00 / 5:30 p.m.–6:30 p.m.	dinner with toddler
6:30 p.m.–7:30 p.m.	bath and bedtime routine: brushing teeth, putting on pj's, reading stories, all the hugs (both parents).

7:30 p.m.–9:30 / 10:00 p.m.	dinner and catching up with husband, maybe watch some TV or do laundry
10:00 or 10:30 p.m.	sleep

So, yeah. Some days are jam-packed with working, and the only time I have with the kiddo is bath time and bedtime, but then the next day I have quality time blocked out for me and my little guy. On very rare occasions, there is a day I don't get to see my kid at all. Those are hard. And there are definitely days (usually once a week right now) where I do not work at all. These are designated family days, and they are wonderful. Sometimes these are filled with adventures, like a trip to the aquarium and a meal in a restaurant (what?!), and sometimes we spend a lazy morning at home and stay in our pj's, followed by a family grocery run and dinner together back at home. These days are always work-free, and I get to focus my energy and attention on me and my family. I also try to carve out some "me time" after the little one goes to bed—maybe I have a nice Epsom salt bath and listen to music or a podcast, or maybe spend an evening under the covers watching my favorite shows that have piled up on my DVR. (With snacks!)

If, like me, you are not a naturally organized person, it may be even more helpful to try to create and stick to a schedule to find your balance. You can set reminders on your phone that will tell you exactly when it's time for the next task to begin. Or if you thrive on a kind of chaos that only you understand (also like me), you can leave yourself sticky notes or take the time to make a to-do list before you go to bed at night. If (unlike me) you are a morning person, you can do this when you first wake up. Your work schedule might be a bit flexible, but you'll soon discover the value of keeping your baby on a schedule for your sleep (and sanity.)

Once you have figured out how to maintain your current work-home schedule, you can start thinking about how to move forward and start adding to your plate. When you're ready, you should feel empowered to ask for more responsibilities or opportunities at work.

Gina, a licensed marriage and family therapist from Redondo Beach, California, shared her story of how she was able to move up and advance her career after returning from maternity leave after having her second child.

"I was back to work by early September, and they posted the management position in November. I knew I'd be good for it—I was licensed, had management experience, and it would take me out of the field which ultimately is safer as a mama. It included a good salary bump, and since I planned to stay at this agency for the long run I knew I had to move up. I talked to my husband first, as it would be a huge commitment. I was currently working four days a week and would have to go back to five, I'd be on call 24/7, and would have crazy hours sometimes. But he said go for it!

I applied and had the scariest interview of my life with ALL the managers and directors at my agency. They later told me how surprised they were by me and that I had applied. I did my job, my work was good, I always hit my productivity, and didn't need to be micromanaged. I got the job and transitioned right in! It was terrifying at first, but here I am now . . . five years later!"

If you feel up for the challenge and have a support system that will help you go for it, then go get that promotion. Always be clear with your employer or supervisor, and don't forget about the "mommy track" they may have subconsciously put you on, assuming you might not be up to the task.

Show them you're ready for more by being consistent in your work, taking initiative, and putting in the time. Only you will know when you are ready to make that next big step. It's your move to make.

EMBRACING CHANGE

Your priorities can change in ways you never expected. You might find yourself wanting to push ahead and advance your current career, or you might want to keep your job but take a step back to spend more time at home, or you might change careers completely. There's no wrong answer.

Here's one mother's story about a complete shift in priorities that led to a brand-new career:

> *Kara, a former retail manager from Brooklyn, NY:*
> *"Before I had my daughter, I wanted a career in the field of architecture, design, or planning, as I have a professional degree in architecture and a master's degree in urban planning. I had only been in New York for a year, and I spent that time interviewing and networking. Additionally, my position at Pottery Barn connected me with some private interior design clients. I really felt like there were so many opportunities. I was so excited! I was committed to myself 100 percent. I worked about 40 to 50 hours per*

week and still found the time to explore the city, see shows, meet with friends, and take dance classes.

When my daughter was born, I knew I would not return to retail/manager work. The schedule was unpredictable and the hours were long. I needed a job that flowed with the normal workweek so that I could maintain a healthy, steady schedule for me and my family. I was just so in love with my daughter, I started to think, 'How can I make money and still be with her?' The answer to that question came in the form of a job working at a prestigious preschool in Manhattan.

All of my decisions were made out of a deep need to remain close to my child. I took a big risk, but within a month, I was promoted, given a substantial raise, and offered tuition remission for my daughter to attend one of the best preschools in Manhattan! A spot opened up for her quickly and she started day care when she was nine months old. We covered half of her monthly tuition costs, and the school paid for the rest. I gave one of my paychecks away, and paid bills with the other.

The feelings of anxiety and worry faded once my daughter was in a preschool program one floor below me. It took some time to get there, and looking back it really amazes me that all those transitions were made at the same time.

If you find yourself in a position where you have to go back to work, consider a part-time return to the workforce or change jobs completely. There is no wrong choice. Stay at home, return to work, work from home, change careers, do whatever feels right for you and your family."

Kara's daughter is now eight years old, and the family has since relocated to Michigan to be close to relatives, but Kara still loves working in the preschool setting, where she is now in a more senior administrative role. Her "temporary" priority shift turned into a new career path.

PART 1 WRAP-UP

Congratulations, new parent! You've made it through part 1. And I'm not just talking about the first three chapters of this book. You've worked your way through the first part of your transition back into the workforce, while doing some much-needed reflection and making some difficult decisions about what you want. Now, it's time to lay the groundwork for how you will make

it all work—and you will make it all work *for you.*
I promise.

In the next two parts of the book, you'll find the tools and information you need to empower yourself to crush all of your goals, both at work and at home. I'm not a psychologist or a life coach. I'm not Oprah. And I'm not your mom or BFF. But I'm a working mom who has experienced my fair share of anxiety, guilt, and discrimination, and I've somehow managed to find happiness and a path forward in a career that works for me and my family. I don't want any other new moms to have to suffer in silence, stifle their ambition, or doubt their potential for greatness. Let's get this. I've got your back. (And in the next part, I'm going to help you figure out what to do with your front!)

Part 2 dives right into the nuts and bolts of breastfeeding, pumping at work, and all the physical and emotional aspects of going back to work while breastfeeding. If you've decided breastfeeding isn't right for your family, or you aren't able to breastfeed—you can skip part 2 and move right ahead to part 3 on page 97 for more thoughts (and facts!) on successfully navigating parenthood and your career.

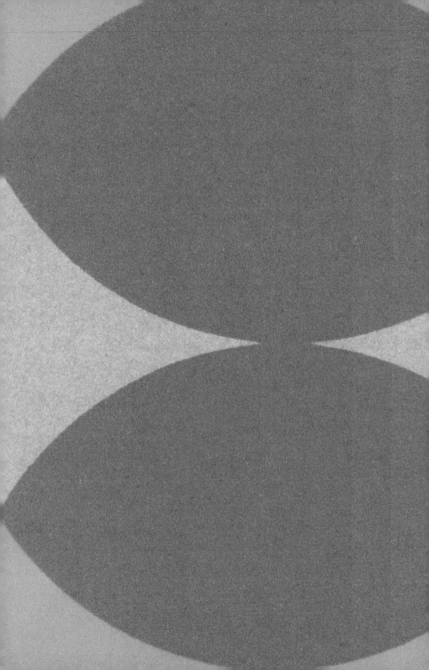

MAMMARY MANAGEMENT 101: MAKING MILKING WORK AT WORK

Welcome to the boob section! First of all, if you are reading this section and are about to go back to work, chances are you have now been successfully breastfeeding for two to three months. So, congratulations on getting this far! I know from experience that it's an amazing thing to be able to do for yourself and your baby, but it can be incredibly difficult and stressful. Luckily, there are ways to prepare for the new challenges of navigating work while feeding and pumping.

If you are not currently (or planning on) breastfeeding, go ahead and give yourself a break and skip this section. You don't have to compare yourself to other mothers or your parenting choices to anyone else's. And whether you're feeling anxious, curious, guilty, or even a little bit jealous, take a minute to remind yourself that you have absolutely made the right choice for you and your family. Nobody here is judging, so neither should you.

Now that I've got your attention, breastfeeders, it's time to talk lactation at work. It's not always going to be easy or comfortable, but you are doing it and you're not alone. Let's make sure you have the tools you need to completely rock this. Because YOU ARE A ROCK STAR.

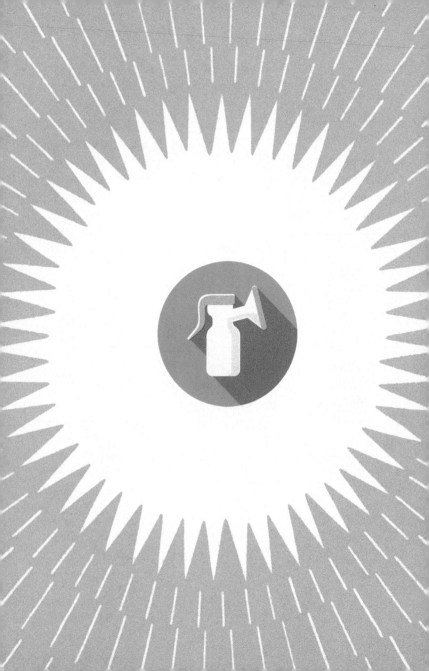

CHAPTER 4

Pump It Up

Welcome to the wonderful world of breast pumps. You might already be a pumping champ, or this might be completely new to you. Either way, we've got a lot to discuss.

Aside from the necessities of having to pump at work to keep up the supply for your baby's demand, pumping can add a lot of flexibility to your life. Some of you may have been pumping since birth, especially if you had an NICU (neonatal intensive care unit) baby. That breast pump can be your best friend if you are producing more than your baby needs in a 24-hour period, for leaving the babysitter a stash to feed Baby while you have (gasp) a date night with your partner, or for pumping and dumping when Mama wants an "adult" drink to take the edge off. It's also a great way to let your nonlactating partner participate in feeding (and for you to sleep through the occasional middle-of-the-night feeding).

But we're here to talk specifically about pumping at work. So let's get to it, shall we?

PUMP BASICS

Not all breast pumps are created equal, and you'll soon figure out what types of pumps work best for you. There are two main types of breast pumps on the market—manual and electric. Within those two categories there is even more variety, including battery operated, hands-free, double breast pumps, and hospital-grade pumps. So, yeah. You're pretty much covered for any type of pumping situation or preference.

Though manual breast pumps offer a lightweight, relatively low-cost option, you will be doing all of the work to produce and collect your milk. Manual pumps are generally held over your breast with one hand while the other hand manually pumps the milk. Overall, manual pumps are a good option for backup or emergency use.

With electric pumps, you get a little more freedom and efficiency, and most standard personal pumps are covered by your health insurance under the Affordable Care Act (more on this later). Personal electric pumps are pretty much the go-to for moms who need to pump at work. You simply plug them into any standard wall outlet, attach them to yourself (you can get a single or double pump), and start a-milkin'! Hospital-grade pumps are generally preferred by and for moms who have multiple babies, damaged nipples, or a low supply of milk. Hospital-grade pumps are a bit more expensive, so they are usually distributed as renters.

If you're looking to multitask while pumping at work or at home, you can get a hands-free pumping bra. This device holds the collection bottles and suction devices in place, leaving your hands free to type, scroll through your Instagram, or feed yourself some snacks. Because, YAY SNACKS.

THE ACA HAS YOUR BACK (AND YOUR FRONT)

Good news: As long as you are covered under any type of private or commercial health insurance, the Affordable Care Act (ACA) has you covered when it comes to breast pumps and pumping at work. The law currently does not cover Medicaid or WIC.

Equipment: Under the ACA, the law requires non-grandfathered insurance plans to cover the rental or purchase of a breast pump at low or no cost and in accordance with what your doctor recommends as medically appropriate. For more information, visit Healthcare.gov/coverage/breast-feeding-benefits.

Education and support: The law also allows for prenatal and postnatal counseling by a trained provider. This includes access to comprehensive lactation support and counseling at no charge. So, if you have questions or need support or advice about making the transition back to work while breastfeeding, please see a Board Certified Lactation Consultant. It's your right.

Facilities: This one is so important. The law requires employers with 50 or more employees to provide mothers with "reasonable break time" in a private space, which is not a bathroom, to express milk until their baby is 12 months old. Companies with fewer than 50 employees should also follow these guidelines, unless they can prove that doing so would create a hardship.

BOTTLE BASICS

Now that you know about the different types of breast pumps, guess what—there are even MORE options to wade through for bottles and nipples. I know, it's a lot. You might be the kind of mom who needs to research and try every bottle and nipple type out there until you find the perfect match, or you might (like me) be the mom who has already made enough decisions for a lifetime, and just goes with the type of bottles you got at your baby shower from your experienced mom friends. If your baby rejects that nipple, you might try another. You'll figure out what works in your own way, with help from that tiny nipple critic you birthed.

In many cases, your baby's feeding patterns will help you determine what type of bottle you need. Some babies who have been exclusively breastfed for a longer period might be more successful with a bottle and nipple that intends to re-create the shape and feeling of a human nipple. Babies who tend to be a little more gassy might do better on a bottle with a filtration system. You and your partner might also have preferences on bottle shape and size; after all, you're going to be holding that bottle in your hands a lot, and your comfort is important, too.

It's also important to talk to your pediatrician and to pay attention to your baby's growing needs over time, as there are different nipple sizes that help control the speed and volume of the flow of milk from bottle to baby. In general, most nipple brands will offer an average of three options: slow flow, medium flow, and fast flow. Sometimes the levels of flow are named or even numbered, with one being the slowest flow.

It seems like a lot of technical information to keep track of and consider, but honestly, it's mostly about instinct. You'll know what's working and not working for you and your baby. The feedback is pretty immediate, if you know what I'm talking about.

ANTARCTICA'S GOT NOTHING ON YOU: BUILDING A FREEZER STASH

We all have that one friend. You know, the one who loves to tell anyone who will listen how easy and magical breastfeeding was or is for her and how she produced so much milk she was able to store away gallons of that liquid gold in her freezer.

And you know what? Good for her. And if that is also true for you, great job, Mama! But not every new mom is a nursing or pumping pro from day one. I certainly wasn't—and I never became one. So take the recommendations ahead with a grain of salt, and if you need help, please reach out to a lactation consultant.

Since I'm not a lactation consultant, I reached out to International Board Certified Lactation Consultant Chrisie Rosenthal, co-author of *Lactivate!: A User's Guide to Breastfeeding*, to give you some pro tips on building your freezer stash and getting ready for that office-pumping life.

By Chrisie Rosenthal BS, IBCLC, RLC

The ideal time to start pumping and storing away some milk in preparation for going back to work is approximately four to six weeks before your return-to-work date.

It's recommended that moms have approximately 20 to 30 ounces of breast milk in the freezer before they return to work. You'll need enough for the first day, plus a little extra so you're not cutting it super close.

The most common way to create a stash is to insert an extra pump session each day and send that milk straight to the freezer. Tip: You'll probably get more from morning pump sessions.

Other ways to create a stash include:

- Start using a Haakaa while you breastfeed. It's a manual breast pump with a silicone milk collection cup that serves as an easy way to collect extra milk.

- Insert a "power pump" sometime during the day, and send that milk straight to the freezer for your stash. The typical schedule for power pumping is to pump for

10 minutes, rest for 10 minutes, pump for 10 minutes, rest for 10 minutes, pump for 10 minutes.

- If your pumped volumes exceed your baby's bottle, you can put the extra milk toward your stash. For example, if your baby takes a three-ounce bottle but you pump four ounces, each time you pump put one ounce into your freezer stash.

- Extend the length of your pump session by 5 to 10 minutes to capture a little extra milk to save.

- Using a hospital-grade pump (such as the Symphony brand) or using the "hands-on pumping" technique will often yield more milk when you pump.

- Combining some or all of these methods.

The closer you are to an oversupply of milk, the more careful you need to be about the extra pump session. A mom with a very strong supply may only be able to do an extra pump a couple times each week, whereas a mom with a low supply may be able to add two or three extra sessions per day and not have a problem. Obviously, watch out for sore nipples when you increase pumping.

The standard schedule for pumping while at work, assuming an eight-hour workday, is to pump both breasts for 15 minutes every three hours. This works out well because Baby should be getting a three-to-four-ounce bottle every three hours. Ideally, your pumped volume from your three pump sessions each day is covering the baby's three bottles while you are away. If you are not pumping enough to cover your baby's bottles, reach out to a lactation consultant to discuss increasing your supply.

Pumping both breasts for 15 minutes replicates a breastfeed. As long as your baby is getting a three-to-four-ounce bottle every three hours and you are pumping every three hours, you are both on the same schedule and your supply will remain steady.

Okay, so you're pumping at work and you're bagging or bottling all of this precious liquid gold. Now, where do you store it? What's the best way to make sure it stays good throughout your commute?

You can store your milk in two-to-three-ounce portions, in either collection bottles or milk storage freezer bags. If your employer-provided pumping room does not have a refrigerator, some moms choose to store their milk in an insulated cool bag in the break room or kitchen refrigerator. Nobody needs to know what's in your flowery lunch bag! (I prefer polka dots myself.) As long as the milk has been kept cool, it should be fine to transport it with you in a cool bag for your commute; just make sure you put it right back into the refrigerator when you get home. Cooled or chilled breast milk is safe for your baby to drink for three days. And don't worry too much about that commute, even if your cool bag isn't the coolest. Room temperature (68 to 72 degrees Fahrenheit) milk is safe for 6 to 10 hours. So, feed that milk to Baby first.

To be extra safe, you can remember the 5-5-5 rule (the numbers are a little conservative, but it's a handy tool to use). The rule is simple: Breast milk is safe for 5 hours at room temperature, 5 days in the refrigerator, and 5 months in the freezer. 5-5-5.

List of Pumping Supplies

- Breast pump—standard, hospital-grade, or manual

- Nipple guards

- Flanges

- Collection bags and bottles

- Cooler or insulated cool bag

- Bottles and caps

- Cleaning supplies

- Nipple shields

- Nipple lube or coconut oil

- Hand sanitizer

- Nursing bra

- SNACK FOR MAMA

- Smartphone or tablet and earbuds or headphones for entertainment

MENTAL HEALTH CHECK-IN: MILK-DRENCHED EMOTIONS

How you holding up, new parent? Hopefully better than I was at this stage.

Your emotions might be all over the place at this point, and that's perfectly normal. Breastfeeding itself—and the postpartum period—causes a constant flow (which sometimes feels like a tidal wave) of hormones, and it's really important to check in with yourself and your mental health before returning to work (which will bring a whole other set of emotional and mental challenges). Your breastfeeding relationship with your baby is about to change in a major way, especially if you've been breastfeeding exclusively and pumping is new to you.

When you breastfeed, your body releases oxytocin, a hormone that reduces stress and anxiety and helps you bond with your baby. Weaning, and even supplementing (which is a completely safe and healthy choice), can abruptly decrease the amount of oxytocin released, leaving you in a sort of withdrawal state. And, of course, less oxytocin means you'll experience higher levels of anxiety and sometimes even feel detached from your baby.

Add exhaustion and everything else that comes with preparing to get back to work, and you might find yourself a bit out of sorts. If, however, you are feeling more than just the "baby blues" or weaning anxiety, please refer to the "Mental Health Check-In" sidebar in chapter 1 (page 26) and don't be afraid to reach out for help.

Therapy is a great resource for new moms. Check with your employee benefits or insurance provider to see what resources they cover. You can also reach out to a new mom support group in your area; these groups are a wonderful way to connect with other moms both online and in person.

Medication, if needed, doesn't always have to mean the end of breastfeeding. Talk to your psychiatrist, physician, and pediatrician to make sure you are taking care of your needs and Baby's needs safely.

And remember, deciding to supplement with formula or to stop pumping or breastfeeding altogether is NOT a failure. Your emotional health is paramount to your baby's development, health, and safety.

If you are in crisis, you can call the National Suicide Prevention Lifeline at 1-800-273-8255. You can also text HOME to 741741 to reach the Crisis Text Line for immediate help.

Find more information at Postpartum.net.

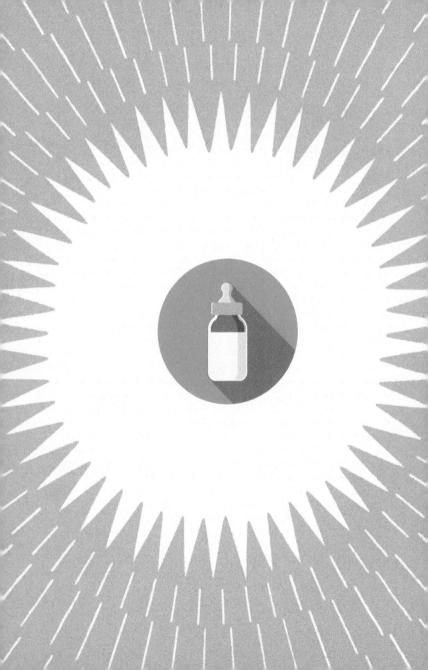

CHAPTER 5

The Boob Olympics: Keeping Up with Your Baby's Breast Milk Habit While Working

You probably never imagined that so many people would take an interest in what you're doing (or not doing) with your breasts now that you're a mom. From family members to friends (with and without kids, even) to the neighbor you just met while you were out on a walk with your newborn, who just had to make small talk by asking if you were breastfeeding, everyone seems to have an opinion on what should be a very personal choice. And now, you're taking the road show to the office. Good times.

Going back to work is going to be a huge adjustment, for so many reasons. That lovely schedule you've got your baby on for sleeping and feeding? Yeah, that's probably going to change. Or maybe you have let Baby sort of set the guidelines for when they want to eat, sleep, or play. Totally cool, but also about to be so different. Bonus: By some cruel joke of fate, the time when most moms have to return to work—about 12 weeks—just happens to perfectly line up with a pretty common fourth-month sleep regression in babies. Who needs sleep anyway?

I know it sounds overwhelming, but I promise it won't last forever. You will find a new schedule and new patterns that make sense for your family, and they will eventually become your "new normal."

TO MAINTAIN YOUR SUPPLY OR NOT: THAT IS THE QUESTION

Now that it's becoming clear that your sleep schedules and feeding patterns, among other things, are going to be shifting, there are some new choices to make. These decisions are important because they can impact your supply and how much breast milk you're giving your baby, and whether you want or need to start supplementing—which is a very safe and often practical option.

Here's some general guidelines for maintaining a supply in various breastfeeding or supplementing scenarios. These are general guidelines from Chrisie Rosenthal, our resident IBCLC (International Board Certified Lactation Consultant), but you should speak with a lactation consultant (LC) or your family physician to make a plan for your individual needs and goals.

For exclusive breastfeeders, pumping every three hours for about 15 minutes while away from Baby will help keep up a full supply. You shouldn't need more than 20 to 30 ounces in a freezer stash. Basically, you should be replacing what your baby eats every day while you're apart.

If you're having a tough time keeping up with pumping every three hours or not getting enough

milk when you pump, then supplementing with formula might be a helpful choice or even a necessary
one. It's important to work with an LC in making
any changes to your feeding and pumping pattern.
If Baby is being combo fed, Mom would typically
continue her routine—subbing a pump session for
when she would usually feed at home. The recommended stash is still pretty much 20 to 30 ounces.

If you're planning on breastfeeding while you're
home and formula feeding while you're at work,
you won't necessarily need to maintain a stash. You
might still pump at work to relieve engorgement.
As always, you should consult with an LC or your
physician before making any drastic changes, as
major shifts to your routine without guidance can
lead to plugged ducts or mastitis.

THINGS THAT ARE OKAY

Just in case it wasn't already super clear, however you decide to feed your baby is 100 percent your choice and your business. However, whether you like it or not, the people around you—especially at work—will have opinions. But you know what? Those opinions do not matter. If you need a reminder, here are some things that are okay when it comes to your work and your breasts.

- Taking the time you need to pump—as often and for as long as necessary. You know what's not okay? Getting mastitis because you didn't feel like you could get away from your desk for 15 minutes.

- Enjoying the time you spend pumping in private at work. Quiet time is at a premium these days, so enjoy it where you find it.

- Hating pumping. It really doesn't have to be your moment of zen. Sometimes, it just sucks. Literally.

- Forgetting to lock the door and getting walked in on. It's going to happen—at least once.

- Forgetting to mute your phone when you're on a conference call and having someone wonder what that strange noise is.

- Forgiving yourself for that noise on the phone.

- Messing around on your phone while you pump. It's your time, and the company is not going to go out of business because you were on YouTube for five minutes watching Kelly Clarkson sing her latest cover.

- Figuring out that pumping isn't for you and choosing to supplement. (You're not alone.)

- Loving your job and not wanting to miss anything.

- Missing a meeting or dialing in, even though it's just down the hall, because you are engorged and uncomfortable.

- Seriously hating to pump.

- Like, hating it a lot.

- Crying during your whole pump session. Remember how we talked about those hormones?

- Missing your baby.

- Calling or texting your childcare provider for an update or photo of your baby. (Sometimes looking at a photo of your baby helps the pumping process. Our bodies are a marvel!)

- Choosing to wean completely. You don't have to prove anything to anyone. Your baby needs a mom who is happy and well-adjusted. It's YOUR body, YOUR choice.

SUPPLEMENTING

First of all, let's get rid of any stigma you may have attached to the idea of supplementing. Banish it far, far away, never to be heard from again. Formula is not the enemy, and it is not a last resort or an indication of a failure of any kind. Supplementing (or even weaning completely) is often a safe, healthy, stress-reducing option— whether by necessity or choice. For me, supplementing after a series of stressful, difficult feedings changed everything. My baby started gaining the weight he needed and we started to connect more. Instead of crying through a feeding, I was able to relax, make eye contact, and be present for my little one. Also, supplementing offers new opportunities for your partner, or any support person you might have around, to help take over some feedings, especially overnight, so you can get some much-needed shut-eye.

You can always talk to your pediatrician for supplementing tips and support, but here's a little primer to get you started.

No matter when you start supplementing, it's a good idea to ease into it. It also helps to do it when Baby is in a good mood. A fussy or sleepy baby might not be up for trying something new, so maybe avoid introducing formula for the first time before bedtime or when Baby is super gassy or cranky.

Once again, I turned to our chief smarty-pants on all things related to feeding your baby, Chrisie Rosenthal, IBCLC, for some general guidelines when it comes to supplementing. It's important to make a plan for supplementing, with support and guidance from your pediatrician or a licensed lactation consultant, and introduce the formula gradually over a few days.

You can begin with one formula bottle for a couple of days and then start to add more formula bottles gradually every two days. Also, not every formula is the same, just like not every baby is the same. You may have to try a few formulas before you find the one that works best for your little one.

There are some differences to be aware of between breastfeeding exclusively, formula feeding exclusively, and combination feeding. First, formula can be a little tougher on Baby's tummy, and tends to be more constipating; however, some babies can and will go back and forth between breast milk and formula without issues or any cause for concern. Second, formula will usually keep your baby full for longer than breast milk since formula takes longer to process in Baby's body. Whereas the volume for breast milk bottles stays steady at three to four ounces after three weeks, formula bottle size will increase over time. With formula, you will need to use bigger nipple sizes on your bottle based on your baby's age, but with breast milk, the nipple size might need to be changed slowly and gradually, or not at all, as the increase in speed and flow of the breast milk might remain at a slow flow the whole time the baby is bottle or combination feeding.

A refresher from chapter 4: The law requires employers with 50 or more employees to provide mothers with "reasonable break time" in a private space, which is not a bathroom, to express milk until their baby is 12 months old. Companies with fewer than 50 employees should also follow these guidelines, unless they can prove that doing so would create a hardship.

The law applies to any nonexempt employees covered by the Fair Labor Standards Act (FLSA). This includes full- and part-time employees who are paid hourly and are eligible for overtime pay (time and a half for any work over 40 hours in a week). Even if you work part-time or have never been paid overtime, you could still be considered a nonexempt employee.

TSA GUIDELINES FOR MOMS WHO HAVE TO TRAVEL FOR WORK

Breast pumps

Traveling with a breast pump does not have to be a stressful situation. The TSA guidelines allow you to bring a breast pump on board in a carry-on bag or suitcase as well as in checked baggage. It can also be carried on as a separate personal item and stowed under your seat. You can contact the airline before you travel to let them know if you plan on pumping in-flight. They might be able to make special accommodations for you or give you some helpful recommendations for your flight plans.

You can also call ahead to your hotel and ask for a refrigerator in your room for storing your pumped milk.

If you're traveling with a breast pump, then it's probably pretty likely that at some point you will be traveling with expressed milk. First of all, don't worry—you don't need to have a child with you in order to carry on breast milk. Since breast milk is legally considered liquid medicine, you are permitted to carry on more than three ounces.

TSA 3-1-1 Liquids Rule Exemption (from TSA.gov)

Formula, breast milk, and juice in quantities greater than 3.4 ounces or 100 milliliters are allowed in carry-on baggage and do not need to fit within a quart-size bag. Remove these items from your carry-on bag to be screened separately from the rest of your belongings. Ice packs, freezer packs, frozen gel packs, and other accessories required to cool milk are allowed in carry-ons. If these accessories are partially frozen or slushy, they are subject to the same screening as other liquids.

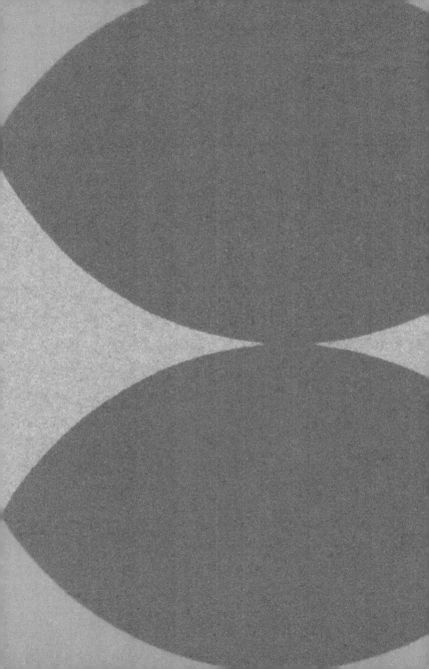

PART 3

FINDING BALANCE AS A WORKING PARENT (OR AT LEAST LOOKING FOR IT)

You've made it to the final part of the book, and now it's time to dive into what life as a working parent is going to look like for you. As I'm sure you're starting to figure out, everything is different now. During your pregnancy, no doubt you made a lot of plans—for how your birth would go, how you wanted to feed your baby, and how and when you wanted to get back to work. One of the most important aspects of parenthood that you're already discovering is the need to adapt and be flexible, because things don't always go exactly as planned.

You can take steps to prepare yourself physically, emotionally, and mentally for all of the changes ahead. This part of the book is all about setting yourself up for success, which might mean something different for you than it did for your sister or your friend, and it might be different from what you used to think success looked like. You'll be provided with the tools to help you find clarity about your working parent goals, to build yourself a support system, and to come up with your new normal at home and at work.

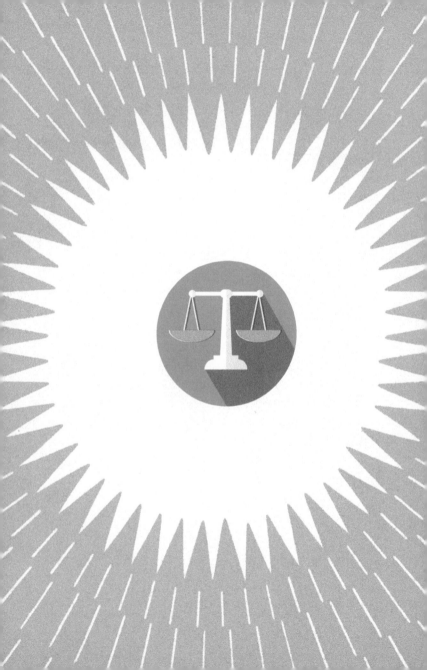

CHAPTER 6

Embrace Your Inner Momager

I t's not a trite sentiment to say parenthood is a job. It's the straight-up truth. You might not be the boss at your other job (the one you get PAID for), but you should definitely consider yourself in a management position at home. You have a lot to juggle and supervise, and you are responsible for staying on top of all communications and research—like reading this book and knowing your rights.

Always remember that you are in control of how you handle your work-life balance and can make adjustments as needed, and with the support of your village at home and the guidance of your employer. I know that sometimes we don't have the privilege of a lot of choices; for some, working long, strenuous shifts in an inflexible environment is necessary in order to survive. Hopefully, you can find not only ways to cope, but also your own power and strength to thrive.

NO MATTER WHAT YOUR CAREER LOOKS LIKE, YOU'RE A MIDDLE MANAGER NOW

Keeping up with the demands of your job while taking care of your own rights and needs as a parent will require a lot of initiative and creative problem-solving on your end. But there are ways to make it easier on yourself. Going back to work equipped with an understanding of your rights in the workplace, the expectations of your supervisor, and your responsibilities to anyone who reports to you, is critical to making your reentry to your career path as smooth as possible.

If you plan on pumping at work, give your employer a heads-up. They might not already have a dedicated space for pumping, but you can give them notice so that they can make the proper arrangements. Remember, this is your right, and advocating for yourself is not asking a favor; it's simply proactive communication.

You can also inform your employer of any needs that have come up in your physical recovery. If you are having mobility concerns due to any childbirth complications or postpartum issues, you can make advance arrangements to work remotely, if possible. This is especially important if you work in a physically demanding job that requires you to be on your feet for hours at a time or to lift and move heavy objects. Take the necessary steps to protect yourself and to give your employer the time to make any possible accommodations.

Knowing your rights and being your own advocate is one of the most important things you can do for yourself as a working parent. While I was still recovering from an emergency C-section, I developed pancreatitis caused by gallbladder stones. The symptoms were incredibly painful (with some bonus nausea), and I wound up having to have my gallbladder removed less than two weeks before my scheduled return to work. If you're keeping track, that's two abdominal surgeries in less than 16 weeks. My return date was not flexible, so I had to make it work. I definitely had some difficulty with mobility, but I was unable to work remotely for the first week back. I was still able to advocate for myself by letting my employer know about my recovery and concerns, and negotiated to get a parking spot much closer to the building. Honestly, that helped a lot. When my physical pain was too much for my commute, I was able to work remotely. So, make sure you can communicate effectively with your manager or your HR department, and ask for what you need, as big or as small as that might be.

For many moms, the last thing you want to be thinking about when you're on leave and enjoying bonding time with your sweet little babe is work. But it might be worth checking in periodically to make sure that both you and your employer are on the same page for your eventual return. If you're feeling like you might not be able to jump right back in and take on all of your former responsibilities at once (and don't necessarily want to get "mommy-tracked"), having clear communication with your work contact is important. This is the time to let someone know that your job is still important to you, as is continuing on the career path you've been on, but that you might need some grace time to ease back into the flow of things.

On the flip side, if your legally protected time off is constantly being interrupted by colleagues or managers checking in to "ask a quick question about that one project" or for any other work-related issues, you should feel empowered to say no. This is your time. The law is there to protect you, and you have every right to disconnect from the workplace while on family leave.

It's all about clear communication.

MANAGING EXPECTATIONS (YOURS, THEIRS, EVERYONE'S)

One of the greatest kindnesses you can do for yourself right now is manage the expectations of your family, friends, and colleagues. Let them know where you are and what you're capable of and ready for, and if you need any time, space, or help. Asking for what you need is not a sign of weakness. In fact, it's a sign of strength and will empower you to get what you want and need in order to succeed.

You should also communicate with your employer about your status and what you need. Remember, you are still recovering physically and emotionally from a life-changing event. (You know, the one where you gave life to another human being?) If your employer is open to it, you can try coming in for a day or two for the first week, just to dip your toes back into the water and get up to speed with what you've missed. Having a day or two back in the office to catch up on emails, technology upgrades or changes, and any workflow changes, as well as getting to know new staff members, can make it a bit easier to come back full-time the following week, feeling more confident and ready to jump in.

Another option, especially if you have someone at work that you really trust, is to ask someone to keep notes for you. They can track any workflow or policy changes or any other information that might be helpful for you upon your return. You can ask them to email you a few times over the course of your leave or have a catch-up meeting with you on your first day back to get you up to speed.

At home, you absolutely should be honest with your partner and the rest of your support team about what they can reasonably expect from you, and what you need from them in order to survive this time. You might ask them to manage a meal train because cooking is not an option for you right now (due to physical or time issues), to help with feedings (especially for parents of multiples), or to just give you breaks from Baby so you can rest. Being open and direct about what you need is the best gift you can give yourself right now.

HOW MUCH SHOULD YOU REALLY SHARE WITH COWORKERS? (OR THE INTERNET?)

If you're anything like me, you probably already have more photos of your baby on your phone than all of your childhood photos (which are tucked away in some box in your parents' garage anyway) put together. What a time to be alive, when we can literally capture every coo, every baby giggle (or baby fart!), and every cute outfit with the touch of one finger. We can video chat with relatives who don't live close enough to come meet the little one in person. Technology has afforded us wonderful and miraculous ways to keep our friends and families updated on our daily lives—the good, the bad, and the stinky. But it's often not just our dearest loved ones who are paying attention. Yeah, in the same way it was so easy for you to find out that the person your bestie is dating puts pineapple on their pizza, with a simple swipe your coworkers, managers, and the person who interviewed you for your dream job can basically see your whole life.

For some people, this is a nonissue. Maybe you work with lots of people with kids who frequently share cute kid stories and parenting frustrations. In that type of culture, sharing some of your own stories might not only be safe, but encouraged. Maybe sharing a story or picture here and there on your public social media profiles might help you bond with that one manager you previously had nothing in common with. If so, awesome!

As with everything on social media, you should use caution about what kind of information you share publicly and how often you share it. You could be subjecting yourself to unwanted and often unintentional or subconscious bias at work. If you post about how overwhelmed you are in your parenting journey, even just in a small moment of exhaustion at home, it could potentially influence opinions at work on your ability to handle a workload. Even if you're only sharing the good stuff—baby's first giggle or those cute fuzzy pajamas that make her look like a bunny—it might affect your professional image, as unfair as it might be. On a personal note, you're also opening yourself up for random parent shaming from Internet strangers who love to judge and criticize even the most seemingly harmless post. The harsh comments or unsolicited advice can take an emotional toll and ruin something that was meant to be joyful.

And once you're back at work, you should be extra judicious about what you share publicly. You might call in sick one day or stay home to take care of a baby with a high fever. If you happen to post a cute photo, someone with baby bias or the person covering your shift might assume you decided to play hooky and spend the day frolicking about with your babe.

Plus, you never know what other people are going through. One of your coworkers or even someone you report to directly might be struggling with fertility issues. You don't have to walk on eggshells, but in a professional environment, try to be sensitive when it comes to talking about your pregnancy, your bonding with your baby on leave, or how hard it is for you to leave your baby at day care. It might be difficult for some people to hear about.

But . . . those fuzzy pajamas are awfully cute, and they really deserve to be seen. I'm not telling you to pretend your adorable, perfect, genius baby doesn't exist. Don't hide that sunshine from the world! It's important to keep friends and family, especially those who are far away, updated with photos and milestones. One way to safely share your baby's life is to create a dedicated private account on your social media platform of choice. You can control the privacy settings, allowing only people you know, love, and trust to have access. This allows people who want to see and hear every little thing Baby does to opt in freely, so you never feel like you're oversharing. It also protects your baby's privacy, which is important because the Internet is forever. Yup. Using privacy settings means when your precious child grows up and starts dating, applying to colleges, and interviewing for dream jobs, they will be protected from their future employer (or high school archnemesis) finding those bubble bath pictures or that video of them shoving a jelly bean up their nose (and the emergency room photos that follow).

So share away, new parent. Just share wisely and be careful out there.

PREPARE FOR AWKWARD ENCOUNTERS GALORE

There's no way around it, there's going to be some really awkward moments as a working parent. If you're still in the breastfeeding stage and pumping at work, prepare yourself for just about anything, from someone accidentally walking in on you to your boobs leaking through your nursing bra and right down to your shirt in the middle of a team meeting. IT'S FINE. I wish I could tell you the number of times I showed up to work feeling bright-eyed and ready for the workday, only to notice halfway through the day that I had baby spit-up on my brand-new work dress THE WHOLE TIME. Pro tip: Always bring a spare outfit and maybe some wipes to work, just in case. Think of it as your own personal diaper bag, because depending on where you are with your recovery, yeah . . . you might also need some form of adult diapers, giant pad, or a change of underwear. (But rest assured—you're not alone in this.)

Remember how we talked about not over-sharing at work? Well, even if you are the most private, discreet person on Earth, you're still going to be hit with super uncomfortable moments with coworkers, neighbors, friends, and strangers. Seriously, you're about to find out that everyone all of a sudden has a vested interest in your bodily functions once you have a baby. It's incredibly weird and often intrusive. I remember one time, when I took my infant son out for an afternoon walk around my block, a neighbor I had never met before walked over to say hello. Literally 10 seconds after we introduced ourselves to each other, she asked me if I was breastfeeding. I mean, can you imagine any other scenario where you would feel okay asking another human being (and a stranger at that!) about what they are doing with their bodies? Like, "Oh, hey, Carol, who I never talk to but just ran into outside the restroom—did you just poop? Was it a good one?" Or, "Hey, Steve, how are those hemorrhoids treatin' ya these days?"

Since we're on the topic of bodily functions, other common yet unexpected moments you might (i.e., probably will) experience at the office include crying for no particular reason (thanks, hormones!) and peeing yourself a little, maybe after a good laugh with a coworker or a sneeze in the conference room, or just because it happens randomly.

Just know that you will encounter some sort of cringeworthy moment(s) when you go back to work. Try to take it in stride and know that you are not alone. And always, always have a change of clothes. (Always.)

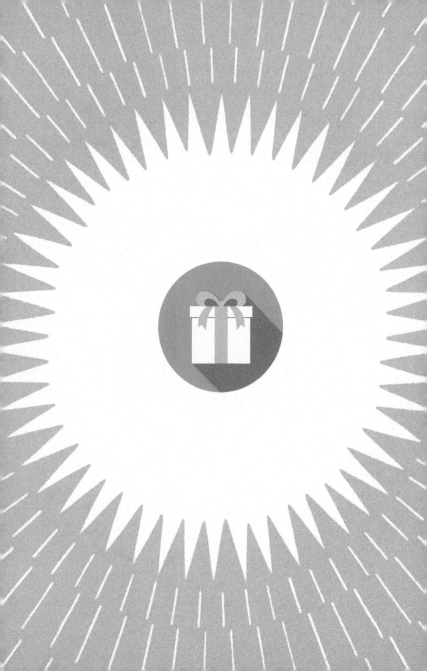

CHAPTER 7

So, Do I Have It All Yet?

For years, Hollywood movies have been selling the idea of "having it all" under the guise of empowerment. You know the scene: A flawlessly gorgeous executive in her perfectly pressed suit and Louboutin heels shines in the boardroom (or operating room) and then comes home, has a beautiful, wholesome meal with her precocious children, reads them all bedtime stories, and gives them advice about that thing they're struggling with (with her makeup fully intact and not a hair out of place) and then still has time and energy for a glass of wine by the fire with her equally gorgeous partner. It's well-intentioned (mostly), as a way to show that women can do all of those things and do them well. But at what cost? And what are we leaving out?

How about the nanny (or stay-at-home parent) who picked up the kids from school, helped with homework and probably cooked that wholesome meal? We need to see the struggle to understand that although it's possible to have all of these things, you can't be everything to everyone all of the time.

Here's the thing—you can do it; you can make it work. You'll start to trust your gut about what the important work things are that can't be neglected, and what can be delegated to someone else so that you can make it home for the things in life that matter the most. It's a constant, ever-changing balance. With a set of clear priorities, a trusted support system, and—let's be honest—a bit of caffeine, you can have all that you want and need to feel successful. And you don't have to lose your own identity (or become a Reese Witherspoon character) to do it.

WAIT, "IT ALL" IS A LOT, HUH?

When a successful woman in almost any type of career, who also happens to be a mother, is interviewed, the first question is always, "How do you do it all?" Yet nobody asks Dwayne "The Rock" Johnson (father of three) or Mark Zuckerberg (father of two) how they manage it all. Either way, the truth is simple. They don't—no one does. At least not without help.

Actor, comedian, and author Amy Poehler has been a very outspoken advocate for domestic workers. When she was honored in 2011 as one of *Time*'s 100 most influential people, she used her speech to acknowledge that having it all means having outside help.

" . . . I thought who besides Madam Secretary Clinton and Lorne Michaels have influenced me? And it was the women who helped me take care of my children. It is Jackie Johnson from Trinidad and it is Dawa Chodon from Tibet, who come to my house and help me raise my children. And for you working women who are out there tonight who get to do what you get to do because there are wonderful people who help you at home, I would like to take a moment to thank those people, some of whom are watching [your] children right now, while you're at this event. Those are people who love your children as much as you do, and who inspire them and influence them and on behalf of every sister and mother and person who stands in your kitchen and helps you love your child, I say thank you and I celebrate you tonight."

You don't have to be a superhero or celebrity to be a good mother or to do well at work. I have had a few days here and there where my kid got a perfectly balanced, Pinterest-quality dinner, followed by some quality crafting time before our bedtime routine. More frequent are the cut-up hot dogs and mac 'n' cheese, followed by some quality time with an iPad or some extra time with our beloved babysitter. Just as there are days where I've been at the top of my game at work and then banged out a whole chapter of this book after my kid went to sleep, there have been just as many days where I showed up, put in the bare minimum to get by, and fell asleep on the couch after picking at my kid's leftover dinosaur nuggets. Or days when my husband and kiddo are having fun in the backyard while I'm upstairs in my home office writing and missing out on all the fun.

Having it all means having the good days right along with the tough ones. It means working late and feeling really good about your role in that project, but not getting to say good night to your little one. It means staying up all night when your baby has a fever of 103.6°, and still going to work, exhausted, the next day. It means finding the rare occasion when you have the time, energy, and money to get a babysitter and have a date night outside of the house with your partner, or a night out to catch up with friends. And it means falling asleep with spit-up in your hair and not caring because your baby said "Mama" for the first time.

EVALUATING WHAT "IT ALL" LOOKS LIKE TO YOU

So what does "it all" mean to you? Take a moment to reflect on the priorities you set for yourself back in chapter 2 (see page 34). You can use that as a foundation to build a vision of what success will look and feel like for you. Maybe work is not your top priority, but more of an obligation that you need to fulfill in order to keep the lights on and feed your family. That's a good thing to know, because having it all might simply mean putting in enough solid effort and time at your current job, or finding something less demanding than your pre-kid career, in order to focus your time and energy on your family. Maybe work is a creative outlet for you, so your perfect balance involves spending your days with your kid(s) and building your online business or writing that novel or making custom orders for your Etsy store—at night or on your own schedule.

And yes, you can still be a great parent if work is a top priority for you! It's okay to love your job and be a boss at it. Your "all" may include leaning on your spouse, family, or outside help. Building a village of people who love and care for your children also makes you a great parent. Working longer hours and missing an occasional bedtime story, but having the financial resources to plan an amazing family vacation once or twice a year, is just another way of loving and taking care of your family.

And there's so much space in between. You can like or even love your job and want to spend time with your family and also have time for yourself. It will take a bit of juggling and (again) a great support system, but moms (and dads!) have been doing it for generations.

One very important thing to do is set clear boundaries both at work and at home. Make it clear at work (as much as your situation will allow) that your off time is yours. Turn off your work email, and let coworkers know not to expect off-hour replies from you. When you are on the job of course you give your best, but as soon as you clock out, try to leave it all at the office, even if the "office" is just another room in your house. The same boundaries can apply to your home life. If you are in a workplace that requires your undivided attention, let your caregiver know that although you might appreciate photo and text updates (which you can look at on your breaks or when the time is appropriate for you), you cannot get any unexpected calls or respond to any messages unless it is an emergency situation.

Another thing to consider is that you're not just juggling work and quality time with the fam. It's not a matter of "do this project or snuggle with Baby." Sometimes, especially in the first few months back, you're going to have to juggle work obligations with parental obligations. Babies—even healthy ones—have a lot of doctor appointments in the first two years. Like, A LOT. And if, like me, you have a child with any kind of special needs, you will need to establish some flexibility in your schedule for visits with specialists and in-home services.

I'm not going to lie to you, it's a difficult dance. But once you set clear boundaries and map out what your needs and wants are at this very unique time in your life, you'll find you learn the steps like a pro. You can have everything you want and give your family everything they need, even if sometimes it's not all at once.

A good exercise to help you create a vision for your career that incorporates your family time is to make a list of goals—both for your career and for your home life, including self-care. You might be surprised by how it might shift some of the priorities you mapped out in chapter 2 (see page 34), or how easily the two lists come together. Write down your goals and then map out what actions you need to take and what boundaries you need to set in order to get there.

YOU ONLY GET ONE BRAIN, DON'T LET IT RUN AMOK

You've figured out your priorities and set your goals. That's HUGE. Your road map might look very different from someone else's—even someone you really admire. THAT'S TOTALLY NORMAL. Do not waste any of your precious time or brain space comparing yourself or your choices to anyone else's, even that seemingly perfectly put-together mom you follow on Instagram or the hilarious "hot mess" mom whose jokes about her kid keep you chuckling on Twitter. Stand secure in what you want out of your life (for now), knowing how much thought you put into the decisions you have made.

It's not a contest. Know that when it comes to your own family, you always win. If having a live-in nanny isn't something you wanted (or maybe wanted but couldn't afford), you don't need to be jealous of the friend who does have one (even though that's a completely normal feeling to have.) It's not what's right for your family. And you don't have to feel guilty (again, a normal feeling) for not volunteering for as much work travel as your colleague who is also a parent. Maybe she wanted more time away and travel is her method of self-care. You can be confident that the work you do and the contributions you make to your team are enough. But also, if you're that mom who *does* want to travel more and needs some space and distance once in a while, you can feel good about that. Your mental health and happiness is a direct factor in the happiness and well-being of your children.

There might be a day when you show up for work exhausted because your baby didn't sleep at all the night before, and you find that your coworker (who is also a mom) is working remotely. You might think, *Ugh, I wish I could be home right now seeing my baby and working in my pajamas*. But maybe she's working from home because she doesn't have anyone to take care of her kid that day and she is super stressed and wishes she could be in the office, focusing on the work. Choose instead to be grateful for the person who is caring for your baby while you get to sip on that mid-morning coffee and dive into a new project.

And please, I beg of you, take everything you see and read on social media with a grain of salt. In fact, use the whole damn saltshaker. Sure, you might find some really cool recipes, crafty projects, and other great parenting tips on Pinterest, but know you don't have to have the most perfectly theme-decorated nursery with a curated array of books and award-winning Montessori toys. Please don't compare your life to someone else's (highly edited) Instagram story. You have no idea what kind of epic meltdown that wide-eyed and smiling toddler had two seconds after that photo was taken, or what *Exorcist*-level projectile vomit that baby unleashed after eating that absolutely gorgeous, organic, homemade puree. Consider how much the apparently glowing, has-it-all-together mom may actually suffer from postpartum depression or anxiety. People have so many ways of trying to cope. We are all just doing the best we can, every day.

Give yourself a break and know that you are doing your best, and that's all your baby needs. Happy parents mean happy kids. Remember when I said that childcare is a form of self-care? It also works the other way around. Taking care of yourself is the only way you can take care of your child.

Each day, try to take a few minutes that are just for you. I know it's hard. "Free" time is at a premium. Whether it's listening to some feel-good music or a podcast you love during your commute, finding a few minutes during the workday to step outside and breathe in some fresh air, or using a mindfulness app to help slow down your breath when you are anxious: You've gotta do you.

THINGS THAT ARE OKAY

Between working, spending time with your family, and taking care of yourself mentally and physically, you now have zero time to give to parent shamers. And no matter what you do, sadly there will be someone in your life or your online feeds who is there to make you feel bad about your choices. Do NOT feed the trolls.

Just to remind you, here's a small sampling of things that people get shamed for that are totally and completely fine, even wonderful. Please don't let anyone gaslight you into thinking otherwise.

- Not going out for drinks after work because you're exhausted or still breastfeeding, or just would rather go home

- Going out for drinks after work. (See! It's okay either way!)

- Keeping your breast milk in the fridge at work. As long as it's sealed and well-labeled, it's perfectly FINE.

- Making your own baby food from fresh fruits and veggies

- Buying canned baby food

- Telling your trusted work friend about your rough night with a sleepless baby

- Not wanting to talk about your baby at work

- Asking the sitter to stay a little longer so you can take a hot shower or a relaxing bath, or even a nap

- Leaving your breast pump on your desk. You have breasts. Your breasts make milk. Your grown-up coworkers can handle seeing the milk machine.

- Traveling for work and not being with your baby for a few days. (Nobody has EVER shamed a dad for this.)

- Sleep training

- Co-sleeping

- Going home as soon as the clock hits 5:00 p.m. (or whatever time your shift ends)

- Volunteering to stay late to finish a project

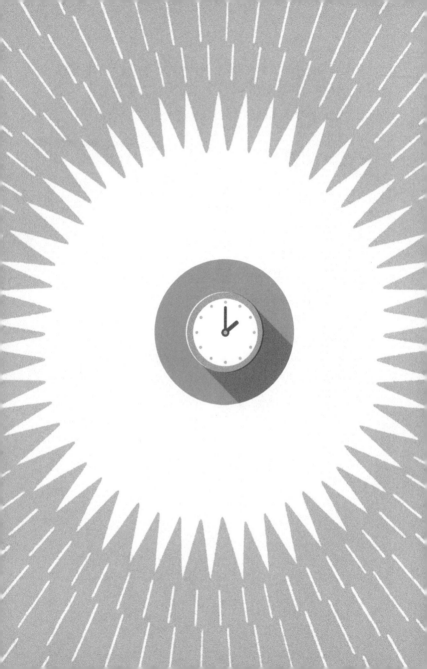

CHAPTER 8

Working 24/7
Isn't What Makes
You Valuable (Not
Anymore, Anyway)

Think back on the early days of your career (or working life if you don't have one main career focus), and on how much you threw yourself into it all. Maybe you were fresh out of school and excited to put all that fancy book learning to good use. Perhaps you had an aha moment that pointed you in the direction toward a shiny, new career goal. Or maybe you just needed to start making money to live an independent life of your own. Either way, it's pretty much universal that those early working days meant putting in a lot of time and energy to prove your worth and forge a path forward.

You may also be feeling like starting a family seems like a whole new career, and you're going to have to put in some long hours and a whole lot of energy. Real talk: Your value in the workplace is no longer just about logging the most hours and putting in the face time. You've got experience and now a very unique skill set that includes multitasking, prioritizing, and delegating. You're about to bring a whole new meaning to work-life balance by realizing just how valuable you really are.

THE "WORK 'TIL YOU DROP" DAYS HAVE ENDED—WHAT'S YOUR NEXT PLAY?

Whether you're going back to your previous job or starting something that fits into your new circumstance, you're going back changed. The wisdom and experience you bring to your company or current project far outweighs your ability to simply "put in the time." You are worth more than the numbers on a timesheet at the end of a week. You've gotten to a certain place in your career (yes, even if you're starting over) because of your own set of unique strengths and experiences. Even while you were on leave, you were making yourself better and more prepared for the work ahead.

Parenthood is all about trusting your own instincts and knowing how to make important decisions under highly stressful circumstances. Multitasking? You are now a boss at multitasking. You could teach a class on multitasking while also feeding your baby and doing a load of laundry. And delegating responsibilities and tasks? You are the expert of delegating at home, and that is going to be an essential part of maintaining balance when you go back to work.

You can trust your gut on when it's okay to put work aside for the day. You've earned it.

Let's try something. Take out a piece of paper and write down the five, (or more) most valuable assets and skills you bring to your job. Really give it some thought and give yourself the credit you deserve. Okay, now that you have your list, take it to heart. Focus on these strengths on those nights when you feel obligated to stay late or go for drinks after work just to prove your loyalty or your worth. I know that sometimes it's hard not to feel left out or behind the times when you hear coworkers reference an inside joke from that thing you missed. And if you have the energy and actually want to participate in after-hours stuff, go right ahead. But if you feel like you have to miss being "in the loop" at home so that you can get some face time with the boss after business hours, remember your list and all of the reasons why the quality of your work matters more than the amount of time you spend trying to make an impression.

WHAT DOES "OFF THE CLOCK" EVEN MEAN?

Whether you work a salaried office job or an hourly gig, work from home or commute into town, work overnight or in retail/service industry shift work, you are allowed to put work aside and be present at home when you're not actively scheduled. In fact, it is incredibly important for that work-life balance we keep talking about and striving for. Since you're so experienced now at setting your boundaries in the workplace, it's time to set some boundaries at home, too.

Have a discussion with your partner about when you might need to be available for your workplace during "off" hours and when your partner might need to do the same. Then, find some solid chunks of time when both of you are able to completely shut out work. Turn off emails, notifications, and put away work phones, laptops, or any other devices that keep you on the hook. Of course, you are allowed to make exceptions for absolute emergency situations, but otherwise, it's imperative to your home life to be able to be present when you're home.

This can be a little tricky for those of you who work from your home. In big contrast to those who head into a main office or shared work space, a home office can often feel like a sanctuary from the messy, loud, and frenetic world that is the rest of your house when there's a baby on the loose. Make an effort to use whatever space you have set up as a work space for just that: for sitting down and doing the work, making the art, filling out those spreadsheets, whatever it is that you do when you're working. If you need some time for self-care or quiet reflection, find a nonwork space for that. Keep yourself balanced by making a clear distinction between "work" and "home"—even when they are both where you live.

This doesn't mean that you can't or shouldn't talk about work at home. Your home is your shelter from the storm, your safe place where you can be your truest self. Lean on your partner or your friends and family when work obligations or stressors start getting to you. Vent. Go off on rants, plan the thousand creative ways you would quit if you won the lottery, curse out that one meanie from the seventh floor—get it all out so you don't carry it with you. On the flip side, share your success stories, gloat about the big commission, do a happy dance because you got some well-deserved praise at work. Tell that funny story about what happened on the elevator or share the hot office gossip with your partner. It's okay to bring home the parts of your day that inform your state of mind. It's okay to enjoy it. It's also totally okay to not want to talk about work at all. Just make sure that when you're at home, you can be fully at home, and not expected—by your boss OR YOURSELF—to be working for free on your own time.

Go ahead and binge-watch that show everyone's talking about already. The laundry will get done eventually. And if it doesn't, you can always buy new underwear. Some parents are Pinterest parents, but it's okay sometimes to be the order-online-last-minute parent.

HOW TO MAKE YOUR EVENINGS AND WEEKENDS COUNT

Remember weekends? Or sleeping at night? Every baby is different, but I promise you at some point your baby will sleep and you will find your stride and be ready to actually get stuff done or—gasp!—leave the house on the weekends. Look, you've been scheduling feedings, keeping track of poops, maybe even making a spreadsheet or two for Baby's intake and output, and now you're managing your work calendar as well. How about scheduling out some time for you to live your life?

Remember the boundaries that you have already set at work and at home. Work with your colleagues to establish the norm that certain days and times are off-limits. Barring literal everything-is-on-fire emergencies, these are the times when you will not be reachable or reasonably expected to respond to messages.

For outside contacts who might not know the ins and outs of your schedule but might send you low- to mid-level priority messages or requests during this time, you can set an email auto-reply letting them know that you are out of reach and what your expected response time will be. You can direct them to somebody with a higher responsibility level or pay grade than yours in the case of an emergency, or just respond if and when you can.

Okay, so you're all set up with boundaries (yay!). Now you've got to stick to them yourself. The world will not collapse around you if you go to the zoo with your family for a few hours on a Saturday. You will not lose your job for having a weekend date night with your partner. (And if you do, then that job is clearly not the one for you—or maybe call a lawyer because that is seriously messed up.) And for the record, date nights are not just for the lucky ones who can swing a Saturday night babysitter. Pizza and a movie in pajamas counts as date night in my house.

If you are like me, you might need some help separating your work life from your home life. I sometimes find myself checking my work email while I'm outside on a walk with my toddler. I don't even realize I'm doing it half the time. One day, my two-year-old actually said, "No more work, Mommy," while we were playing with Play-Doh. Ouch. Luckily for us, there's an app for that. There are actually several apps out there to help you shut out certain functions on your phone and force yourself to be present. You can block work notifications to social media so you can focus on enjoying your day of fun instead of comparing it to some "influencer" mom's curated day of fun, or you can simply put your phone in "do not disturb" mode for a couple of hours.

In general, try to do what you can to be fully present when you're home with your baby and your partner. Enjoy the snoring, sleeping baby on your chest while you try to eat a sandwich. Revel in the giggles and drool-filled smiles. Monday morning is just around the corner and you'll be missing that undeniable scent of the top of your baby's head. That email can wait.

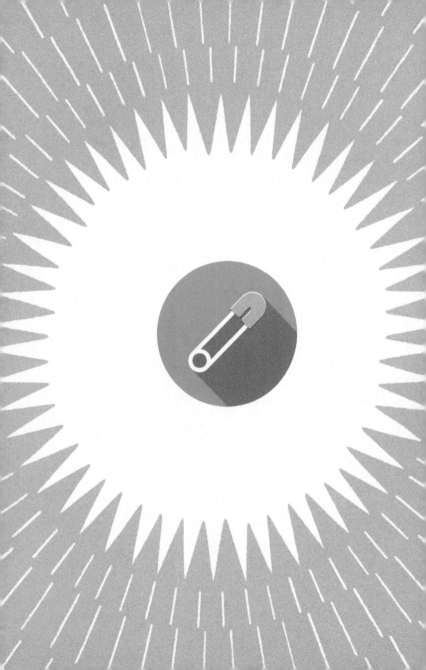

CHAPTER 9

A Support System: Why You Need One More than Ever

Now that you have mapped out your goals and priorities, you might be starting to realize that you need some help in order to put your plan into action. You *can* do everything and have it all, but you can't do it alone all the time. Beyond any childcare arrangements you have made, you are going to need a support system to lean on when life gets busy or overwhelming.

There's not one right way to build your team, just as long as you have some people you can trust and depend on. For some, it's immediate family members and their partner. Others reach out to friends. Some of us are even lucky enough to have the kind of friends who we consider our chosen family. Some find new, enduring friendships in support groups for new moms, both online and in person. For me, and for many other new parents struggling to make it all work, an important member of the support team is a therapist. And don't forget about support at work. Who's that work friend who always has your back? Having them is going to become more important than ever.

THE 10 QUESTIONS YOU AND YOUR PARTNER/ SUPPORT SYSTEM SHOULD SORT OUT EARLY

1. **How you will divide and cover late-night feeds**

    Coming up with a clear plan for scheduled night feeds is going to be so important for your ability to get the rest you need for work. Making (and sticking to) the plan will eliminate any middle-of-the-night games of "rock, paper, scissors" or exhausted arguments over whose "turn" it is. If you are exclusively breastfeeding, this might be a great time to start introducing pumped bottles so that your partner (or any other live-in support person) can take some of the load of getting that baby fed while you get some rest.

2. **Scheduling childcare drop-offs and pick-ups**

    Unfortunately, most childcare situations outside of your home don't exactly cater to your work schedule. Set up a schedule ahead of time with whoever is going to be helping get your kid to and from day care. It's helpful for you AND for Baby to keep to as regular a schedule and routine as possible. Sure, there will be some exceptions. Maybe you typically do the morning drop-off on your way to work, but need to call in a favor every once in a while for an early-morning meeting. Knowing who is available and willing to help on a consistent basis will make life a whole lot easier once you're back in the swing of things.

3. **Emergency and sick day protocol**

Schedules and routines are great, but there's always going to be the unexpected fever (babies get sick all the time, especially in day care), or other random emergency. (Once, my child's day care was being evacuated due to wildfires nearby.) Make sure you have worked out with your partner or other support person and your childcare provider what the emergency or sick child protocol will be. Who should the childcare provider call first? Is it the parent or family member who works and lives closest to the care center and can get there fastest? Is it the parent with the less demanding work schedule who would most likely be able to drop everything? Who are the backup emergency contacts (i.e., the people you trust to pick up your child under urgent circumstances)? Also, work out the logistics, such as: Do these backups have a car seat? Do you need to get them one? These are questions best answered now, instead of in the middle of a crisis.

4. **Budget**

We talked about setting a budget for childcare way back in chapter 1 (see page 16). Now is the time to really sit down with your partner (or with a professional financial advisor or online budgeting planner) to make a general budget for your day-to-day work life. Raising a child is expensive, and those midmorning coffee breaks and restaurant lunches add up. You may need to tweak your routine a little bit from your previous work experience. Maybe bring your own lunch to work a few times a week to help balance the financial load. Try to make a weekly or monthly budget that covers everything from fixed expenses (e.g., mortgage or rent, childcare, utilities, diapers, etc.) to flex spending and saving (e.g., work clothes, lunches, family vacations, date nights, etc.).

5. **Setting boundaries at home for work and off-hours communications**

   Take those "off the clock" boundaries we talked about earlier and put them into action. Set specific times when phones and other work devices are put away or silenced. You can also set times when it's okay and appropriate for checking in with work or doing some work remotely, but make sure that when you are in a designated "off" time you can just be present with your baby, your partner, or friends and family who might be there for you.

6. **Expectations for housework, cooking, and more**

   Whether you are on this parenthood journey with a partner or by yourself, it's a good idea to set reasonable expectations on what needs to be done around the house and how it will get done. If you have a partner, you can divide up household obligations. Or if you can afford to compensate your nanny or a separate housekeeper for an additional duty, acquire help that way to make sure everything gets done. If you're shouldering the load on your own, it's time to take your friends and family up on their blanket "if you ever need anything" statements. Ask for help. Maybe ask a trusted friend to set up a meal train where friends and family can pitch in by bringing over a home-cooked meal on a set night of the week, or even give you gift cards to restaurants that deliver. Maybe that friend who is dying to come over and catch up can also help fold laundry or hold the baby while you do some dishes. It's great to have these things figured out as much as you can BEFORE things start to get overwhelming when you are back to being a full-time employee AND a full-time parent.

7. **Backup plans (including pediatrician number, backup babysitter, etc.)**

Even when it's not an emergency, sometimes plans change. It's a good idea to have a list of names and numbers handy for any and all people who are part of your village. Anyone who might potentially be hanging with your babe should have more than one way to reach you, your pediatrician's number, and numbers for other backup babysitters or family and friends who can help out in a pinch. This also includes providing information about any special needs, allergies, or other important issues for anyone spending time around Baby.

8. **Love languages (words of affirmation, acts of service, receiving gifts, quality time, physical touch)**

What are your preferred love languages? According to Dr. Gary Chapman, the main five are: words of affirmation, acts of service, receiving gifts, quality time, and physical touch. In the hustle and bustle of working-mom life, things like personal connections and feelings can get lost in the shuffle. Make sure you and your support person know the best way to show your affection and appreciation for each other. Maybe you respond most to quality time or physical touch. If so, you can let a friend or partner know that sometimes you need them to just be there to hang out or give a hug, without having to ask for it. Maybe your person needs to hear actual words of appreciation or receive a small token or gift once in a while to feel appreciated. I'm not talking about priceless jewelry here, but just a little something to let them know you are thankful for them and their help. It's easy to be so laser-focused on the baby and the job that you lose sight of your own emotional needs or ways to express your gratitude for those who are helping you maintain balance.

Read more about Gary Chapman's five love languages at 5LoveLanguages.com.

9. **Self-care**

Now that you and your support person know how to care for each other, it's time for you to figure out how to care for yourself. Have an open and honest conversation, first with yourself and then with whoever needs to hear it, about what you need in terms of time and space for your own self-care. This self-care might be having a half hour to decompress when you get home before taking over the childcare responsibilities, or it might mean having some alone time after the baby is asleep to go for a walk, take a hot bath, or read a book without any interruptions.

10. **Parenting style and choices**

Last, but absolutely not least, is setting clear expectations about how you are choosing to parent your child. It's essential to be completely direct with anyone helping raise your child about what issues and parenting styles are important to you. As we've covered, this can be a tricky subject to broach with Baby's grandparents, but it still needs to be done. Important personal preferences regarding feeding (e.g., breast milk vs. formula vs. combo feeding), sleep training, baby-led weaning, co-sleeping, screen time, etc. should be expressed clearly in order to avoid any major issues or misunderstandings (or unnecessary drama) along the way.

THE FIVE FRIENDS YOU NEED IN YOUR PARENT LIFE

1. **The friend who does the research and knows everything**

Who needs Dr. Google when you have a bestie who always has the answers at the touch of a finger? This is the person who went through everything you're now going through, only a couple years ahead of you, and can help you sort out the ins and outs of everything from picking the number one safety-rated car seat to how to get what you need at work. It's probably the person who gave you this book as a gift.

2. **The friend you can be completely honest with**

   SO important. This is the person you can confide in during your darkest moments. The one you can complain to about your partner, and who will always have your back and won't hold a grudge, because they know sometimes you just have to vent.

3. **The friend who knew you before you were a parent**

   After becoming a parent, it can feel like you've lost a sense of your own identity outside of parenthood. Having that person who has known you forever will keep that side of you alive and well. It's the person you turn to when you need a night out or a good laugh.

4. **The friend who is also a working parent**

   Someone who gets it, who shares your struggles and celebrates your triumphs because they're living it, too. You can be there for each other and commiserate about all of the ups and downs of that working parent life.

5. **The friend who shows up**

   Your bestie, your ride-or-die, your PERSON. Whatever you call them, this is the friend who will always be there when you're in need. The one who would drop everything when you are in crisis, or will call or stop by to check in on you without having to be prompted.

THE FIVE FRIENDS YOU NEED IN YOUR WORK LIFE

1. **The one who already has kids**

   This person will be your ally. You can commiserate with them about the struggle, and together you can make sure your company is taking care of your rights in the workplace. It's nice to have someone else around who would rather get home to their little ones than go out for drinks after a long shift.

2. **The one who makes you laugh**

   Plain and simple, we all need that one friend who makes us laugh and take a break from the weight of the world we are shouldering sometimes. This is the person who will take you out to lunch and make you feel like your old self, which is still in there, and part of your new self.

3. **The one who has your back**

   Who's the one person you know you can tell anything to, without fear of being reported at work? The person who will cover for you when your break goes a little long because you're on the phone with the babysitter, or fill you in on the meeting you missed because you had to take your baby to the doctor? Be sure to lean on this person.

4. **The higher-up who can mentor you**

   This is solid advice for anyone, whether you're a parent or not: Make a connection with someone who is in a position you aspire to be in someday. Let them give you advice and help you set reasonable, meaningful goals. It's a bonus if this person is also a parent who can empathize with what you're dealing with.

5. **The notetaker**

Yup, just like in high school, it's always a good idea to be friends with someone who shows up, takes notes, and generally has their life together all the time. I'm not advocating you find someone you can "use" for your own benefit, but hopefully someone you're already friendly with is the kind of person whose organizational skills help balance you out when there's something you've missed.

PARENTING IN CRISIS MODE

We've talked a little bit about backup plans and one-off emergencies. These are the times when schedules and routines go out the window in favor of "survival mode." In survival mode, you're just trying to get through the day and night. But what happens when everyday life turns into survival mode 24/7/365? With the outbreak of the Covid-19 pandemic in 2020, a lot of parents have been forced into a reality of parenting in a crisis for an indefinite amount of time. As I sit here writing this, we are still self-quarantining with a toddler, and working from home with no childcare. We have no idea when his preschool will reopen or when we will feel safe enough to send him back if it does.

The first rule of parenting in crisis mode: talk about parenting in crisis mode! Seriously, though. Whether it's a global pandemic or a personal family crisis, there are others out there who know what you are going through. Reach out. Ask for help, advice, or just a friendly ear to talk to. Take care of yourself so that you can care for your family.

Remember that survival mode is just that: surviving. Do what you need to be able to get through the day in whatever your new normal is. Give yourself a little bit of grace if your kid is getting more screen time than you'd normally like, or if your child's meals don't look like a perfectly nutritious work of art. Mac 'n' cheese and an iPad can be your best friend in times of crisis.

It doesn't matter if your house is a mess or if you haven't washed your hair in a week. What matters is that you are able to keep yourself and your family safe and healthy. Make plans for how you will get whatever supplies you will need, from food and water to first-aid kits and flashlights (plus extra batteries). Take some time to think about having an emergency prep box.

Be kind to yourself. Find ways to help your children cope. Find someone or something that helps *you* cope. And remember, this, too, shall pass.

YES, IT'S OKAY TO ASK FOR HELP (REALLY, IT'S WEIRDER NOT TO)

A little story: A couple of months after my son was born, I was invited to a lunch outing with some other mom friends. One woman, whom I didn't know before, asked me who was watching my son. When I told her he was at home with his dad, the woman looked at me wide-eyed and said, "Alone? Is he terrified?" To say I was taken aback was an understatement. I truly didn't understand the question. Why would my husband—who is as much a parent as I am—be terrified to be alone with his son? It was then I realized how fortunate I am to have an equal partner in parenting (not a dad who "babysits" his own kids). The more I reached out to other moms as I wrote this book, the more I realized that for so many women, the weight of the emotional, physical, and mental burdens of raising children is theirs to carry. Yes, there are great dads and partners out there helping to shoulder the load, but so many of us feel the need to do it all on our own.

Let's talk about that. Why do so many women feel the need to do it all, and to do it by themselves? Is it a cultural or societal pressure to be the nurturing caregivers? Maybe some women feel like they have a certain vision for how they want things done and feel like the only way to get it done right is to do it all themselves? Is it that we are too proud to ask for help? Or even too afraid to admit we need help, that we might not be seen as "strong" or "empowered" or "fierce" enough?

Well, I am here to tell you that asking for the help you need—from your partner, your family, your friends, and even your employer—is absolutely a sign of strength. It will empower you to be the best version of yourself because none of us is an island. Nobody can do it all alone; remember Amy Poehler's words (see page 118) along with these from fellow moms:

> **Rebekah, a teacher and single mother from Seattle, WA:** *"I asked my sister for help with childcare and she has watched both of my kids at no cost to me, which is an immeasurable help both financially and psychologically."*

> **Ashley, a marketing manager from Burbank, CA:** *"I was about to head back to work and had not really had my hair cut in many months (I enjoyed the heck out of my beautiful, full pregnancy hair—every last strand!). But I was heading back to work and my hair was now starting to fall out in clumps (ugh, post-pregnancy woes). My best friend and "unofficial*

*by blood but official in every sense of the word"
aunt to my children showed up to babysit while I
got my hair cut and colored. My daughter wasn't the
easiest and I was pretty nervous to leave them alone
(where I couldn't rush back) for a few hours. I came
back and my friend and my daughter were lying on
the ground with soft blocks all around. Both had
big smiles. It was such a sweet moment and created their own bond for life—and reminded me that
having helpers is absolutely necessary."*

Whether you are a single parent navigating this
on your own, or married with your in-laws living with
you full-time, it's okay to reach out and ask for help.
All of those friends, neighbors, and family members
who said to call if you ever need anything meant it.
(Well, 90 percent of them, at least.) So, ask for what
you need. You know those friends who are dying to
see the baby? Let them come over and hold that
baby while you take a hot shower—and make them
bring food. Ask for meal trains, rides to pediatrician
appointments, notes from the office, or to have a
friend come over and sit with you when you're feeling alone (even in a house full of people). Anything
you would do for someone you love, chances are
there's someone out there who loves you enough to
do it for you. You deserve it.

How are you doing, new parent? Aside from the chemical and biological changes that happen with the birth of a child, a new baby is always a huge change—and change is *hard*. You should always continue to take stock of your emotional, physical, and mental well-being. It's not enough to check in once and move on. It's a process, one that can evolve as you and your baby change and grow. That's why I'm asking you to check in with yourself here again.

Keep in mind that even if you are handling everything and feeling ready to get back into the swing of things at work, postpartum depression and anxiety (PPD and PPA) can still show up at any time during the first year, and transitioning back to work is definitely a period of high risk. Beyond the "baby blues" or other complicated feelings about going back to work and separating (temporarily) from your baby, mood disorders like PPD and PPA affect more than 15 percent of mothers every year.

If you feel like you are experiencing any symptoms of PPD or PPA, it's so important to reach out for help right away. Your mental health has a direct impact on the emotional and physical well-being of your baby. Studies have shown that untreated maternal mental health issues have a lasting impact on child development. Infants and toddlers of depressed mothers are at greater risk for developing insecure attachment, dysregulated attention and arousal, and difficulties in cognitive functioning and social interactions, according to a study by the Canadian Paediatric Society.

It's often difficult to recognize signs and symptoms on our own, so it might be helpful to go through this section with someone in your life who can help you from an outside perspective. Hand this book over to someone you love and trust to guide you through the PHQ-9 questionnaire mentioned on page 27.

If you recognize any symptoms or feel like you are in crisis or need to talk to someone, contact your trusted health care provider or reach out to a licensed clinical therapist for help.

If you are in crisis, you can call the National Suicide Prevention Lifeline at 1-800-273-8255. You can also text HOME to 741741 to reach the Crisis Text Line for immediate help.

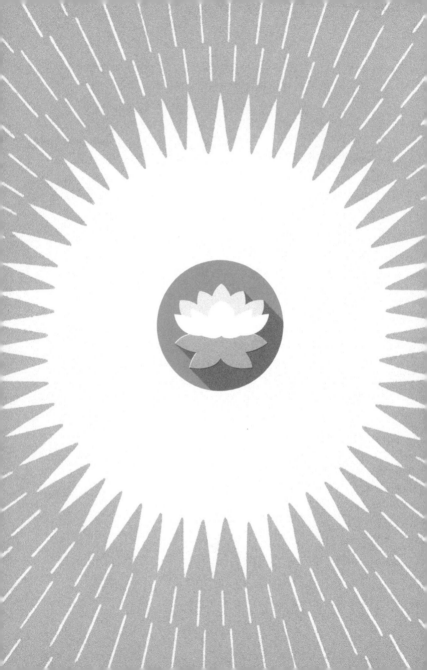

CHAPTER 10

Mindful Momming: This One's for You

This is it. To paraphrase Lady Gaga, you're on the edge of glory! You know how to take care of your baby, how to take care of business at work, how to prioritize the important stuff at home, and now it's time to remember to take care of yourself. Your emotional well-being will directly impact the well-being of your family. But more than that, your well-being and happiness are important because YOU are important. Never forget that you are a whole person—not just a parent, an employee, a partner—and you are just as deserving of care, support, and joy as all the people who depend on you for their care, support, and joy.

What does self-care mean to you? The phrase itself has become a bit of a buzzword, co-opted by social media "influencers" to mean treating yourself to a mani-pedi or a glass of rosé. Real self-care is about way more than that, although those little things do go a long way. I remember taking a long, hot shower while my mom took care of my newborn, and it felt like a whole weekend getaway on a spa vacation. What we're talking about here is really taking stock of your own needs and making sure you take care of yourself—whether that means a nice soak in a hot bath with Epsom salts or a weekly session with a licensed therapist. I mean, RuPaul says it best: "If you can't love yourself, how in the hell you gonna love somebody else?"

Can I get an amen?

One thing that can help new moms a ton is another buzzword: mindfulness. Yet a bit of mindfulness goes a long way. It's worth giving it a try. Here's how it's officially defined:

Mindfulness: (noun) The practice of maintaining a nonjudgmental state of heightened or complete awareness of one's thoughts, emotions, or experiences on a moment-to-moment basis (Merriam-Webster).

What follows are some suggestions for mindfulness specific to new moms. Give these a try when you need some help centering yourself or appreciating the present moment.

MINDFULNESS EXERCISE 1— A MINDFUL WALK FOR TWO

Practicing mindfulness can be a tricky thing when you are looking after a newborn who needs your constant attention. Sometimes you just can't get away, even for a few minutes. But that's okay, because you can use this exercise to be mindful together!

Take a mindful walk with your baby. Whether you prefer to wear your baby in your favorite carrier or show them the world (or let them sleep) in their stroller, that's your call. Leave your phone at home, or at least in "do not disturb" mode if you need to have it with you. First, focus on your breathing, especially after getting yourself together and getting Baby dry and clean, strapped in, covered up, and ready for a walk outside. You might be just a little frazzled, so it's time to slow down and listen to your body. Step outside and take three deep breaths in through your nose and out through your mouth. Really fill up that belly with breath.

Let go of any thoughts about the laundry that needs to be done or the phone call you need to make later. Be fully present and take in the world around you. To you, this is just the same sidewalk you walk or drive past every day, but to your newborn, it's a whole world they have not yet discovered. Walk a little slower. Notice how your feet feel with each step. Feel the warm sun or a cool breeze on your skin. Take note of how quickly or slowly your body is healing from your birth. Keep breathing and keep moving. Talk to your baby about what you see, smell, and hear along the way. You might even surprise yourself with a new discovery or two of things you had never noticed before.

MINDFULNESS EXERCISE 2— HOT BEVERAGE BREAK

Hopefully, you will be able to find even 5 to 10 minutes to spend alone, maybe while Baby is sleeping if you're at home, or during a little bit of downtime at work. Fix yourself a nice hot cup of whatever pleases you. I know some parents can only function at high levels with their coffee fix, and some (like me) prefer a soothing herbal tea (although caffeinated teas are also a good way to get that extra boost for non-coffee drinkers). Some days my hot beverage of choice is simply hot water with a few squeezes of lemon juice. Ah, and there's always hot cocoa in the fall (or really anytime you want—no judgment).

Find a quiet spot that's as private as possible, and settle into a comfortable position with your warm cup of goodness. Hold that cup with both hands and feel the warmth radiating through the cup to your hands, and from the cup up to your face. Close your eyes. Feel the texture of the cup—is it a smooth ceramic mug? Does it have some textured paint or design on it? Any nicks or chips? Bring that cup up to just under your nose. Breathe it in—the steam, and the smell of that divine drink. What sensations or thoughts arise? I know you probably really want to take a swig already, but just pause in this stillness for a moment. Notice what you're feeling. What outside thoughts are running through your brain about work, your baby, or your grocery list? Try to melt away any thoughts that are not about this very simple act of getting ready to drink. Take a deep breath, unclench your jaw, relax your tongue—which you probably didn't even realize you were doing. Relax your shoulders and maybe give your neck a soft roll around once or twice in either direction.

Now, bring that irresistible cup of joy up to your lips and take a sip. Not a gulp, just a sip (seriously, don't burn the roof of your mouth or your tongue—that's no fun). Let it sit in your mouth for a few seconds, and really take in every nuance of the taste and feeling of the warmth on your tongue. Now go ahead and swallow and feel that wonderful warmth trickle down your throat and into your stomach. Take an indulgent deep breath, then go ahead and take another sip. As you drink, try to stay present in this little moment of your much bigger, fuller day. Don't think ahead to the emails that might await you at your desk or the diaper that might need changing. Just. Drink. Your. Tea.

Notice how much longer your drink stays warm. Even when it cools down a bit, is it still satisfying? How is your body changing as you make your way through the cup. Is the caffeine elevating your heart rate? Is it helping you wake up after an exhausting night with a fussy baby? Is it actually relaxing you after a stressful morning meeting? Do you need to pee? Try to take this time for yourself at least once a day. Notice what, if anything, changes over time.

MINDFULNESS EXERCISE 3— SCAN YOUR BODY FOR TENSION, AND RELEASE IT

Here's a simple but effective mindfulness exercise you can practice from the comfort of your own bed. You can do it right before bed or just as you wake up in the morning, or both times.

Lie on your back, or in whatever position is most comfortable or neutral for you. Start with your toes and work your way up your body. How are your feet

positioned? Are they tense or loose? Are you holding any stress or anxiety there? When I'm stressed,
I sometimes hold my toes in a curled position and
don't even notice until I get a cramp. Remember
to take long, deep breaths in through your nose,
out through your mouth. On an exhalation, release
any tightness or tension from your feet. Let your
feet roll around from the ankle a few times until
you come to a relaxing and comfortable position.
Now focus on your legs. Are they straight or bent?
Are they warm under the covers, or cool hanging
out from under the sheets? Are they all tangled up
in that top sheet? Continue your focused breathing and give your legs some attention. Maybe they
need a gentle massage, or maybe they just need to
be detangled and stretched out flat (be careful not
to lock those knees), or even curled up into a cozy
side-sleeping position.

Now move up to your belly. What's going on in
there? Did you get enough to eat, or is your tummy
rumbling for a little snack? Take a moment to think
about your recovery from your birth experience.
Are you feeling any soreness or cramping? Let go
of any anxiety or unwanted tension you are holding
in your belly. Breathe through those uncomfortable thoughts that are making little knots in your
stomach. It might be helpful to keep a heating pad

close enough to your bed so that you can reach out and grab it without much effort. Let your breath truly fill up your belly, and give meaningful, deep exhalations.

Continue this process as you notice your fingers, hands, and arms. Are they lying flat beside you? Are your hands buried under your pillow, giving your head some extra support? Are they holding on to another part of your body that needs some pressure or massaging? Try to bring your hands to a place of rest and unclench any tightness you're holding on to.

Are you still carrying the weight of the world on your shoulders? Channel your inner Elsa and let it go. Let it all go. And finally, focus on that head atop your shoulders. Release any tension in your neck. Give it a couple rolls, clockwise and then counterclockwise. Unclench your jaw and let your tongue sit comfortably, not jammed up against the roof of your mouth. Close your eyes and keep focusing on that breath. Be present and aware of your body in this space and at this moment. What are the last thoughts you have before drifting off to sleep? What is the first thing that crosses your mind in the morning, before you grab that phone and start focusing on that screen? Try to take in all of the positive thoughts and breathe through the negative ones. And just keep breathing.

CONCLUSION

Well, here we are. As you close the final chapter of this book, you are ready to go off and conquer this new chapter of your working parent life. Hopefully this book has helped you organize your thoughts on what you want to accomplish next. But here's the thing: Just like Dorothy from *The Wizard of Oz*, you've had everything you really needed all along. You're a strong, powerful parent who knows what you want and has a plan to put it into action. Your natural instincts and abilities are your ruby slippers. This book was just the tornado that knocked you into your Technicolor world of empowerment and confidence.

Basically, you're a boss. You've always been a boss. So, take a deep breath and get to work. And love on that sweet baby of yours. But don't forget to take care of yourself, too. It's okay to be scared. It's also okay to be excited. You're going to feel all the feelings. Take it all in. This is YOUR time.

And yes, I'm aware that I am about to sound like a sappy Instagram influencer, but you know what? I don't care, because this is the absolute truth: You've got this.

RESOURCES

Flipd. (Flipdapp.co)—Allows you to lock yourself out of your phone for a set period of time and promotes mindfulness.

Postpartum.net
The home page of Postpartum Support International (PSI) offers information, resources, and support for the emotional changes that women experience during pregnancy and postpartum.

Offtime. (Offtime.app)—This app helps you balance digital device usage in your life.

REFERENCES

American Academy of Pediatrics. "Federal Support for Breastfeeding." Accessed May 10, 2020. AAP.org /en-us/advocacy-and-policy/aap-health-initiatives /Breastfeeding/Documents/FederalSupportfor BreastfeedingResource.pdf.

American Academy of Pediatrics. "Returning to Work." Accessed May 10, 2020. HealthyChildren.org/English /ages-stages/baby/breastfeeding/Pages/Returning-to -Work.aspx.

Anxiety and Depression Association of America. "Post-partum Disorders." Accessed May 10, 2020. ADAA.org /find-help-for/women/postpartum-disorders.

Benefits.gov. "Family and Medical Leave Act (FMLA)." Accessed May 10, 2020. Benefits.gov/benefit/5895.

Bernard-Bonnin, A.C., Canadian Paediatric Society, and Mental Health and Developmental Disabilities Commit-tee. "Maternal Depression and Child Development." *Paediatrics & Child Health* 9, no. 8 (October 2004): 575–83. doi.org/10.1093/pch/9.8.575.

Care.com. "The Care Index." Accessed May 10, 2020. Care.com/care-index.

Chapman, Gary. *The Five Love Languages*.
Chicago: Northfield Publishing, 1992.

Crisis Text Line. CrisisTextLine.org.

Healthcare.gov. "Breastfeeding Benefits." Accessed
May 10, 2020. Healthcare.gov/coverage/breast
-feeding-benefits.

Krause, Jill, and Chrisie Rosenthal. *Lactivate!: A User's
Guide to Breastfeeding.* California: Rockridge Press, 2019.

Kroenke, Kurt, Robert L. Spitzer, and Janet B.W.
Williams. "The PHQ-9: Validity of a Brief Depression
Severity Measure." *Journal of General Internal Medicine*
16, no. 9 (September 2001): 606–13. doi.org
/10.1046/j.1525-1497.2001.016009606.x.

Medela. "Breastfeeding Guide." Accessed May 10,
2020. Medela.us/breastfeeding/articles.

Postpartum Support International. Postpartum.net.
Accessed May 10, 2020.

TSA.gov. Accessed May 10, 2020.

US Department of Labor. "Family and Medical Leave
Act." DOL.gov/agencies/whd/fmla. Accessed
May 10, 2020.

INDEX

ACKNOWLEDGMENTS

Eternal gratitude to Justin and Raffi for putting up with my work and writing schedules (which kept me from backyard shenanigans and kitchen dance parties), and for loving and supporting me always.

Thanks to my amazing family for always believing in me and especially to my mom, who made the transition to work a million times easier. Thank you for being the best mom and Nana in the world. You are our rock.

To the caregivers who have loved my son and made it possible for me to work: Sose Simonyan, Alicia Smerk, Candice Morris, and Aislyn Carter—you are my angels.

Love and thanks to my "blue jean baby, LA ladies" for helping me survive that first year: Lindsay, Taysha, Ashley, Andrea, Christine, Katie, Gina, and Liz.

And to my dearest friends, who kept me sane, focused, and laughing throughout this whole book-writing process: Mattie, Jake, Nasti, Susan, Chrissy, Kara, Dani, Tad, and Kristin—y'all are the best.

Special thanks to Chrisie Rosenthal for your wisdom, and to all the women who shared their stories for their honesty and generosity.

And finally to Morgan, my editor and my friend. I'm so thankful for your faith in me and for helping me bring this book to life.

ABOUT THE AUTHOR

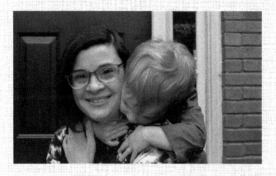

Ali Velez Alderfer is a writer, journalist, and mother who is always trying to nail down that perfect work-life balance. Her work has appeared in *Newsday*, BuzzFeed, and CNN. As a storyteller, she has performed in such series as Tattle Tales, A Very Special Episode, Shine, and the Los Angeles Scripted Comedy Festival. She did her undergraduate studies at Emerson College and obtained a master's degree in education from Harvard University. In her very rare spare time, she enjoys going to the bathroom uninterrupted and eating an entire meal while it's still hot. She lives near Atlanta, Georgia, with her husband, toddler, and two dogs. You can find her on Twitter at @MeAliVelez and follow her evolution as a parent at TheMamaFiles.com.

CPSIA information can be obtained
at www.ICGtesting.com
Printed in the USA
LVHW020425151120
671396LV00001B/1